THE LATINA
GUIDE TO HEALTH

THE LATINA GUIDE TO HEALTH

~

Consejos and Caring Answers

JANE L. DELGADO, PH.D., M.S.

~

Foreword by Antonia Novello, M.D., M.P.H., DR.P.H.
former U.S. Surgeon General

NEWMARKET PRESS

This book is published in the United States of America.

First Edition

ISBN: 978-1-55704-854-7 (English-language paperback)
1 2 3 4 5 6 7 8 9 10

ISBN: 978-1-55704-855-4 (Spanish-language paperback)
1 2 3 4 5 6 7 8 9 10

Library of Congress Cataloging-in-Publication Data

Delgado, Jane L.
 The latina guide to health : consejos and caring answers / Jane Delgado ;
introduction by Antonia Novello.
     p. cm.
 ISBN 978-1-55704-854-7 (pbk. : alk. paper) 1. Hispanic American
women--Health and hygiene. I. Novello, Antonia C. II. Title.
 RA778.4.H57D445 2009
 613.089'68073--dc22

QUANTITY PURCHASES
Companies, professional groups, clubs, and other organizations may qualify for special terms when ordering quantities of this title. For information e-mail sales@newmarketpress.com or write to Special Sales Department, Newmarket Press, 18 East 48th Street, New York, NY 10017; call (212) 832-3575 ext. 19 or 1-800-669-3903; FAX (212) 832-3629.

Web site: www.newmarketpress.com

Manufactured in the United States of America.

～～～

This book is designed to provide accurate and authoritative information in regard to the subject matter covered. It is not intended as a substitute for medical advice from a qualified physician. The reader should consult her medical, health, or other competent professional before adopting any of the suggestions in this book or drawing inferences from it.

The author and the publisher specifically disclaim all responsibility for any liability, loss, or risk, personal or otherwise, that is incurred as a consequence, directly or indirectly, of the use and application of any of the contents of this book.

Contents

⌒Foreword

M Y MOTHER HAS ALWAYS BEEN MY ROLE MODEL. Her life at eighty-six is full of joy, laughter, friendship, and continuous education. I think there is no greater wish for any of us than to model such a life. I may have become Surgeon General of the United States and benefited from the finest of medical education, but it is my mother who taught me common sense and encouraged me to always provide for the common good. Likewise, throughout her life experiences, she has come to understand that health is about much more than medical systems. It is about knowledge, caring, giving, sharing, and choosing to treat ourselves and others as we want others to treat us—basically, *con cariño y respeto* (with affection and respect).

The same answer to how my mother has lived her long life is ours to have. It is in the traditions of our culture, taking the time to care for ourselves, and then doing what is needed to care for others. In a way it is like being a *comadre* (friend) to others and helping them celebrate—in one—life's blessings. There is a great comfort and joy in knowing a true friend, one who is caring and understanding but above all is only a phone call, e-mail, or text message away. I am pleased to have this friend in Dr. Jane Delgado, and as a good *comadre*, I want to share her with you.

In *The Latina Guide to Health*, Dr. Delgado offers a "life package," if you will, where advice filled with common sense is given. In this guide to health, Jane weaves together the everyday stories of character and wisdom of all types of *hermanas* (sisters) and Latinas and then presents the latest advances in science and medicine in a concise, informative, and easy-to-understand format. In this book our stories as sisters, daughters, mothers, wives, and partners are intertwined with love, affection, and truth, a way to show the world that our gender accomplishes the impossible and, most times, there is no one to give us credit.

In *The Latina Guide to Health*: Consejos *and Caring Answers*, Dr. Delgado gives us a caring and tender guide to health from a friend who understands our worries and fears and exposes our strengths. This book is advice you can trust and share.

Life takes all of us on different paths, but we all need a friend on that journey. Jane is one of my life's most cherished *comadres*. I know you will find her guide useful and witty. It is a guide for your journey that will ease your path. Read it, and you will finally have a true friend.

—ANTONIA COELLO NOVELLO, M.D., M.P.H, DR.P.H.
EXECUTIVE DIRECTOR, GOVERNMENT AFFAIRS
WOMEN AND CHILDREN'S HEALTH POLICY
FLORIDA HOSPITAL FOR CHILDREN
FORMER U.S. SURGEON GENERAL

⌒Introduction

THIS GUIDE IS WRITTEN FOR *YOU*—LATINAS OF ALL AGES, sizes, family backgrounds, and family situations. I have spent my whole life working to improve the health of Hispanic women and their families. Today, as never before, there is advice—*avisos y consejos*—for our minds, bodies, and spirits that can help us to be healthier and happier than ever before.

I want to have a conversation with you, as I have had with so many Latinas I have met across the country and the Spanish-speaking world. Just as if we were talking over a *chocolate caliente* (hot chocolate) or *café con leche* (coffee with milk), I want you to know that I am an honest, straightforward person who supports you for who you are while asking you to do the best you can for your health and happiness.

All of us need to hear and remind each other that it is okay to see the world in a different way because we are Latinas. *Aguantando*, our belief that to be good women we have to endure and hold everything together, is important to us. But sometimes we do it too much and end up neglecting or even hurting ourselves. When we have accurate information, when we see the truth, when we value ourselves—along with our families—we discover the hope and motivation to take care of our total well-being.

As the president and CEO of the National Alliance for Hispanic Health, I oversee and manage programs throughout the United States that each year reach millions of people. During the past decade I have watched how many major leaps forward science has made and how much has changed in health care since I last wrote a book for Latinas in 2002. At the same time, the many women who have shared their

It is okay to see the world in a different way because we are Latinas.

⧜

stories with me have told me that their experiences with their own health have not reflected these changes. I became certain that whatever I would write next would build on their stories and my experiences.

I also knew that this book would be different because two of my *comadres* who had been vitally important to prior books for Latinas, Deborah Helvarg and Henrietta Villaescusa, were no longer alive. Both health professionals, they were well informed and not silent, and they had health insurance. Despite these facts, they both experienced the fissures of our uncharted health system. In some of my last conversations with each of them, they made it clear that I had to carry on our mission—their life's work—to improve women's health. They inspired me to write *The Latina Guide to Health* for all of us trying to live our healthiest, happiest life and help our *comadres* do the same. In the stories and advice in this book, I hope I have been able to capture in some small part their love of life, wisdom, and devotion to friendship.

I must admit that while taking care of Deborah, I saw the dramatic shifts in the health care system that had occurred over the preceding decade. Hospitals were glad to have someone (me) stay in the room and help with the care, since they were so short staffed. There were innovative treatments on the horizon; but to get them, you had to meet the strict requirements of the clinical trial that had been constructed to validate the treatment. Cancer treatment was more tolerable, but for lung cancer the outcomes remained dismal. Hospice and palliative care were available; but in order to receive these services, you had to agree to forgo any treatment for your condition.

Deborah reinforced my belief that while science can answer some questions, the body-mind-spirit connection goes beyond the explanations of science. Deborah's enormous desire to spend one last Thanksgiving with her sons and all of us who made up her *familia* (family) helped her beat the odds regarding how long she would live. She died twelve days after a Thanksgiving feast with her sons she adored, plus her friends and other family members.

Making this book meaningful and medically sound took the support, belief, and work of many experts. Dr. Ken Blank (Capitol Women's Care) is a dedicated bilingual obstetrician-gynecologist who gave up his weekends to review every word in this book and provide his knowledge and wisdom. There were also several generous colleagues who reviewed specific sections: Dr. Don Schumacher and Kathy Brandt (National Hospice and Palliative Care Organization), Dr. Jack Lewin (American College of Cardiology), Dr. Martin Seligman (University of Pennsylvania), Dr. Juan Enriquez (Excel Medical Ventures), Sandra Raymond (Lupus Foundation of America, Inc.), and Dr. Sandra Hernandez (San Francisco Foundation). All of these persons brought the best of science and clinical practice to bear while appreciating our reality: for Latinas, health is a complex mix of body, mind, and spirit.

Until recently, little was known about Latina health.

It is not surprising that the information about us is only now emerging. Until recently, little was known about Latina health. In fact, the U.S. government did not even collect statistics on the causes of death among Hispanics before 1989. This means that there have been many assumptions about our health and illnesses that have been based on myths, not facts and science.

In the last several decades, however, research has yielded a wealth of new information that challenges previous assumptions. The bottom line is that we may be healthier than we thought, but we also may be suffering from diseases and moods that may be more preventable and treatable than we previously knew. We do not have to accept either poor health or suffering as part of being Latina today.

The most surprising news is that even though Latinas have high rates of diabetes and are more likely to be overweight than non-Hispanic white women, Latinas have lower rates of heart disease and stroke, and they live longer than non-Hispanic white women, rich or poor.

Yet, there is also news that Latinas' longer lives are not necessarily healthy or happy. We appear to be more vulnerable than other women to certain diseases (e.g., depression, diabetes, and arthritis) that can compromise our quality of life when left untreated.

For example, here are some facts:

- Latinas do have a higher rate of diabetes than non-Hispanic white women. You can take action to delay its onset and prevent the negative consequences of the disease (including the life-altering need for amputation of a leg and loss of vision) with an emphasis on eating healthy foods, increasing physical activity, maintaining a healthy weight, and making other lifestyle changes.

- Latinas are more likely to suffer from depression. Worst of all, for more than a decade the rate of attempted suicide among Latina teens has been the highest of any group. The causes are complex, but I want to motivate Latinas to seek help and, as a consequence, save lives.

- Hispanics absorb certain drugs differently than do people from other groups. Therefore, we must be very careful when taking prescription or over-the-counter medications, as well as alternative supplements and medications.

- Latinas are more likely to develop cervical cancer than other women, yet Latinas are less likely than other women to have regular Pap tests. We cannot let family and cultural history keep us from getting the tests we need. I want to help you understand all your health risks and encourage you to get the tests you need. Avoiding medical care will not make you healthier, but preventive actions on your part can.

- Finally, we come to the emotional and culturally important topic of our weight. According to standard height/weight charts, many Latinas are overweight. But deeper analysis of the research reveals that many of us are built differently than non-Hispanic women, and weight may not be the best measure of health. I will explain how to reconcile these differences and develop meaningful goals tailored to you as an individual, so that you can be realistic about your body.

This book was borne from the stories women have shared with me, my commitment to improve women's health right now and in the future, the science that is unfolding at this very instant, and the need to overcome the flaws in our health system. I know that the time to care for our health is now. While there are lots of new facts about health, they are useless unless there is a fundamental change in how we think about and approach our own health.

Too often leaders in the health community forget what makes people do new things. Facts rarely change people. Encouraging new attitudes and presenting facts that are directly relevant to daily life are what change people, since those steps support people's ability to apply knowledge and make sound decisions.

If you talk to health care providers, they complain about the lack of patient "adherence" or "compliance." I look at many of them and think the real problem may be that what they say is neither compelling nor convincing. I know that when Latinas want to do something, we take care of the *planes* (arrangements) to make things happen. We get strong and we get determined. We speak with our friends and relatives—all of our trusted sources—to find out how to handle whatever we need to do. As Latinas, we listen to each of our stories and learn from each other.

So how do we begin to think about our health in a new, positive way?

So how do we begin to think about our health in a new, positive way? There is so much information to cover. It is no wonder that many health-related books tend to be tomes. They are often filled with admonitions about things to do, things that we know we have no intentions of doing, or discussions that are irrelevant to our lives. What most of us need is to feel safe having discussions about our own health and resources.

When it comes to our health, we must begin to pay better attention to what we need. We need to create an environment where we prioritize taking care of our health and see it not as a chore but rather as something we do because it is good— good for ourselves and our families. We need to acknowledge our fears *and then do whatever it takes to care for ourselves.*

In countless ways we find ourselves in an information age where we are totally wired to each other yet still not able to lead a healthier life. Knowledge and technical expertise are not sufficient. Too often we are unable to blend the parts of health that we *have* to do with the more intimate and individual aspects of what we feel and *can* do. Knowing the facts is a small part of our success, and if we are confused, we should not be surprised. Every day we hear from experts. Too often they remind me of those experts who can tell you ten ways to have better sex but haven't been on a date in years.

To deal well with health care in the twenty-first century, you need to have a *comadre*, a best friend and health care buddy. I was that *comadre* for my dear friend Deborah. I took notes, asked questions, stayed calm (as best as I could be), and helped her get through whatever emerged until the very end. For most of us, we have to be our own *comadre*. With *The Latina Guide to Health* I hope to be one of your *comadres*, one offering information to improve your health.

The Guide reinforces and shares the *consejos* and wisdom of our culture to help each one of us be advocates for ourselves, our friends, and our families. It means we have to learn to rethink each aspect of our health and learn to celebrate our own health.

We begin by examining, in chapter 1, how we see ourselves and how the very strengths in our communities (*familia* and *cultura*) sometimes need to be tempered. Before we can see our health in a new way, we need to see some of our family and cultural beliefs in a different way. We need to recognize the emotional barriers and strengths that affect our attitudes and the way we care for ourselves.

Once we begin to open our minds, we can start to think about the impact of science on our health, the increasingly comprehensive view of illness and wellness, and changes in the patient–health care relationship that require greater knowledge and individual action. We look at all of these issues in chapter 2. To benefit from twenty-first-century medicine, we need to understand what a genome is and why having a gene does not, by itself, determine whether or not you have a specific condition. We all need to understand the concept of risk factors and how to apply it to the choices we make. Most important of all, we need to know how to get the most from our changing health care system.

Building on our new understanding of our cultural legacy and medical realities, we can focus on taking care of ourselves to maximize our health and well-being, as discussed in chapter 3. Having a healthy body means maintaining a healthy lifestyle with exercise, healthy eating, a healthy environment, sound sleep, proper screening and diagnostic tests, and medications when needed (from prescription drugs to aspirin to alternative medicines). Having a healthy mind means more than merely not having illness. Mental wellness is available to every woman today, given all the new treatment approaches (medication *and* therapy) and the recent findings (from the emerging area of positive psychology) about the benefits of nurturing and developing character strengths and virtues. And we all know the primacy of nurturing relationships, sexual intimacy, and faith as key factors for good health.

As Latinas, we also need to come full circle and acknowledge that caring for others in our life—our children, our partners, and our other family members—is another part of our health. As *comadres*, we need the commitment to share the wisdom gained through caring for ourselves and others, and in chapter 4 we explore what it takes to fulfill this commitment.

Latinas are the chief health decision makers in our families and communities, relying on information passed from mother to daughter: a bit of science, a home remedy, and words to soothe the spirit. These strengths need to be bolstered by empowering Latinas to also incorporate the best of science and technology when determining the right health decisions for our own well-being. What we Latinas need most are the *ganas* (determination and will) to apply solid information and practical advice to better care for ourselves.

This is not to say that we should ignore our families or abandon our culture. Far from it. But first, we have to realize that we cannot compromise our own health for the sake of others.

Once our *ganas* have been fired up, we will be ready to apply information from Part Two ("Taking Care of Our Health Needs"), which contains many resources that support our taking action. The information in Part Two's "Essential Facts and Resources for Latinas" focuses on those areas of greatest interest and impact for Latinas and their families. Additionally, this part quickly dispels myths and succinctly provides facts, as well as tips about keeping up with the best and latest resources available online. Part Two also contains a "Glossary of Frequently Used Words." Part Three, "Record Keeping and Resources," provides key tools for organizing and tracking your health information, plus more suggestions about valuable health-related resources.

My mother often said, *"Donde hay vida hay esperanza"* (Where there is life, there is hope). No matter what health issues you're facing, *The Latina Guide to Health* is written to help make hope a reality for you. My sincere wish is that we all may celebrate each day by taking care of ourselves—in body, mind, and spirit.

"Donde hay vida hay esperanza" (Where there is life, there is hope).

17

HEALTH IN THE LIFE OF TODAY'S LATINA

Part One

Overcoming Our Barriers to Health

It was the weekend, and once again I was going to call to catch up with Yolanda. As soon as I got on the phone, I could hear her breathless tone. She was speaking in that voice that meant that she couldn't talk to me now. It wasn't that she didn't want to, but she had too much to do. She had to take her father to the doctor, then take her mother to the pharmacy, take a conference call from her home, and decide what she was going to make for dinner that night. A hardworking woman with several part-time jobs, she was constantly juggling to balance caring for her parents, being there for her daughter, and dealing with the extra demands of a husband who attended only to his work. I asked her if in all her scheduling she had scheduled anything for herself. She laughed as she said, "Of course not—I do not have the time!"

HOW DOES SOMEONE RUN OUT OF TIME? AS LATINAS, WE ARE often stretched to the limit by our obligations to our family, our work, and whatever else is on our plate. Most of these commitments are ones we gladly make, but sometimes our enthusiasm and sense of what has to be done overtake what is reasonable for us to do. We want to be good and helpful, and we believe our families and family time come first. But the speed with which we say yes to others—often before they even ask—distracts us from looking at our own health and well-being.

When we Latinas talk among ourselves, it's obvious that we share feelings of being burdened, stressed, and overwhelmed. The most negative outcome is that our own health and well-being become the easiest items to push off our to-do lists.

But are Latinas really different? Aren't all women overextended? The answer is clear: yes, on both counts.

Multitasking is not new to women. As mothers, we know that the "m" in mother stands for "more than one thing."—Eliana

In many ways we Latinas share much with other women—issues of balancing family and work, the joy of finally getting equal pay for equal work, the need to go for regular breast exams and Pap tests, and so on. Yet even though we share these similarities, Latinas are different in subtle ways that have a huge impact on our lives. We live longer than non-Hispanic women, but we suffer more from diseases that compromise the quality of our longer lives. The stress we experience in our close families, along with our dependence on family, turns one of our greatest strengths into our weakness. As a result, we are good at taking our children for their vaccines and wellness visits, but we do not make appointments to see our own health care providers.

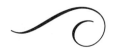

FAMILIA (FAMILY)

WHILE MOST CULTURES CHERISH THE IDEA OF "FAMILY," for us *familia* means so much more. Decades of research support our personal experiences with *familia*. Compared with non-Hispanic women, we are more group oriented, more community oriented, and more "other" oriented in general. The concept of "me first" is not only unappealing but also a sign of being rude and *malcriada* (badly raised).

Does this mean that we are one big happy family? Of course not. Latinas, like other women, struggle with their family members. Some want more autonomy, while others want less. There is no one-size-fits-all lifestyle. Yet we try to come to terms with what our family means to us and the impact they have had on our lives.

The Hispanic culture imposes an enormous sense of the need to have family connectedness, even when relatives are physically far away, relationships have been far from ideal, or there is emotional distance. And when we do not have the family we want, we create new relationships to give us that sense of belonging. Our concept of *familia* is all-encompassing, as it reaches beyond blood relatives to include people who are part of our emotional community. It is a unique way of connecting with others and of nurturing that strong sense of family in our culture.

When we get together, we ask each other about our families, friends, and relationships as we try to see the linkages that may exist. For Latinas, this sense of belonging to a group is important. Our role models are not those Latinas who are solitary and independent but rather women who are connected to others. We like to be—and, for many of us, need to be—part of a family. This is a good thing in many ways. People who are connected to others tend to live longer and healthier lives; they are also less likely to suffer from depression. These are the good consequences of the Latina concept of *familia*—but there are also drawbacks.

What does not help us is the idea that our families are the only people we can trust and depend on. There is a common belief that we should neither discuss our problems outside our close circle nor seek help beyond it. This kind of focus on family goes beyond caring to becoming controlling. It can even entrap us in situations that are unbearable. It is at this point that *familia* generates an emotional chokehold on any action we would take to meet our own needs as individuals.

Doing things for ourselves becomes difficult because of how we set up our priorities. There is much that we convince ourselves we have to do for others. We live as if each day had more than twenty-four hours. First, we take care of our family members and friends, then we meet our job commitments, then we keep our house in order, and finally, we keep our clothes and *cosas* (things) in order. By the end of the day there is only enough time to put on our pajamas, go to bed, and—if we're lucky—have enough time to get a good night's sleep. Then, we start the same cycle all over again the next day. *Familias* may be wonderful, but they can also be exhausting. The question is, How can we balance the love of *familia* with what we can reasonably do? Understanding the need for that balance is an important first step toward our own health. To take care of ourselves, we need time which we often need to claim from others in our lives.

Since those around you benefit from all you do it is also in their best interest that you stay healthy, refreshed, and happy.

Cultura (**Culture**)

Jane, I just don't know how to tell you that we are different. We don't all eat beans. —Carmen

My family has been here for 300 years; my values are different.— Leticia

I have lived in this country for 40 years and I have always felt like a foreigner.— Lucy

EVERY TIME PEOPLE GATHER ON A REGULAR BASIS, THEY create a way of being and interacting. Culture is what we eat, say, do, wear, pray, love, and hate. Culture happens at school, work, church, and communities, and in each of our families. Groups of people create ways of doing things that bind them together. Culture has to do with how we see ourselves and how we relate to others. It includes everything from the language we use to the "right" way to do things.

I cannot tell you how often people confront me about my use of the terms *Hispanic* and *Latina*. Typically they say, "How can you use those words when *Hispanic* or *Latina* is made up of many groups of people that are all so different?" My response is always the same: "The same way we use *non-Hispanic white* or *Anglo*." That we are the mingling of several cultures only enriches who we are.

Whether or not we Latinas admit it, our own mix of cultures affects everything we do. Too often we are made to feel as if we do not belong to the culture that surrounds us. How often are Latinas asked, "Where are you from?" (Reply: "Los Angeles.") Followed by a more emphatically asked, "No, really—where are you from?" (Reply: "My parents are from Arizona.")

Everything from such comments to certain glances to the subtleties of the politics of exclusion and bias steals from us the energy derived from our *sí se puede* (yes, we can) conviction. Too often people look at us, hear our names, or hear us speaking and consider us not to be Americans. Yet Americans we are.

On a recent trip outside the United States, some of the people I met commented that I was a "nice American." That combination of words struck me as unusual because when I am home, my fellow Americans do not see me as an American but as someone who is from somewhere else. And then there was the "nice" part. "Nice," I learned from further discussions, meant that I behaved like someone who valued other cultures, attempted to speak the language, and was polite. Sadly, the typical American is still seen as someone who dresses too casually for the place or setting, speaks loudly, and assumes that everyone knows English.

When I was younger I thought of myself as an English speaker with the ability to speak Spanish. My view of who I was changed when my mother and I went to one of those amusement areas where you play a game and end up winning a little plastic toy. Not being very coordinated, I avoided the games that required shooting or throwing balls. I preferred the game where you would try to toss rings around a wooden block.

As I randomly threw the rings, I was surprised when my last ring toss ended perfectly over the block. I knew instantly that I had won the largest stuffed animal. In my joy I shouted, "¡Gané! ¡Gané!" (I won! I won!) I don't know what surprised me more— that I won or that I announced my joy in Spanish.

At that moment it became clear to me that culture was very complex. I knew that I spoke English 98 percent of the time, but when the moment came to express deep emotions, I did so in Spanish.

—Jane Delgado

We are also affected by changing views of culture and what it means to belong. In the 1980s there was much discussion about the need for persons not born in the United States to adopt and fit into the predominant culture. For Latinas to be successful, we had to go through a process of acculturation. It did not seem like a good thing to me because it meant that in order to be part of the U.S. mainstream, I had to give up my own culture. I was not thrilled at the prospect of having to give up what I wanted to celebrate.

Today, we as a society have evolved to a point where acculturation refers not to a giving up of culture but to an exchange that occurs when different groups work and live together. It refers to communities being able to learn from one another. Consider what defines American cuisine. Although many people still think first of ketchup, that's now outsold by salsa.

But salsa aside, the question for each Latina to answer is, what does it mean to be a Latina in the United States? The answer is simple: it means different things to different people. But that is not the answer people want to hear. Most non-Latinas are looking for an easy way to capture who we are. The mainstream media that are so integral to how we are perceived and how we see ourselves do not capture all our other roles and identities.

The media images of Latinas in television (whether English or Spanish) are both distorted and overly dramatic. The advantage for Latinas with Spanish-language television is that we are cast in all the roles. In the English language media we are usually portrayed either as maids or as hot Latin lovers. Some of us are both; most are neither. We need to look at what is healthy for us and to have role models in all media that look like us.

We are also a large and significant group of women. As of 2009, Latinas account for one in every six women in the

United States. This means that there are as many Latinas in the United States as there are people in all of Australia.

Given our diversity and numbers, we should be a highly valued part of society. Instead, too often we are submerged within the catchall term *minority,* which by its use and implication diminishes our impact and devalues our contributions. Society's devaluing of us dampens the *ganas* (determination and will) with which we need to approach our everyday life and especially our health.

But dampening of our passion is the past, and nurturing our *ganas* is the future.

BRINGING IT ALL TOGETHER

THE CHALLENGE WE FACE IS TO RELISH THE JOYS OF *familia* and *cultura* while releasing the chokeholds on our lives. To take care of our health means that we have to have *ganas* with booster rockets, since health requires our active participation. It is our unique combination of American assertiveness and Latina *respeto* (respect) that will make us successful as we take the actions we need to improve our health.

Since your health and well-being are vitally important, you have to take care of yourself. Remember, it all begins with you.

Making Today's *Medicina* Work for You

WHILE SOME LATINAS DO NOT WANT TO FOCUS ON their own health because they are too busy taking care of their families, other Latinas hope their health problems will go away if they do not talk about them, and still others feel constrained by taboos about discussing one's own health.

At a basic level, we sometimes cannot talk about our own health because we cannot find the words to express what we are feeling. This is especially true when we speak in English. In English *health* refers only to physical health; mental health and spiritual health are left for other fields of study. For Latinas, this makes us not trust the health care system. As one *amiga* (friend) said to me, "How can a health care provider know what is wrong with me if they don't know my feelings and my struggles?"

For many years there was a myth that Latinas preferred folk medicine. In reality, the practitioners of folk medicine were some of the few providers of medicine and health care who were located in the community, and who knew the language and customs. Not only was mainstream health care something physically outside the community, it was also fragmented in its approach. It looked at the health of the body, separate from mind and spirit. As a result, Latinas looked for practitioners who were in the community, spoke the language, and understood the culture. That is how folk medicine found its greatest support.

When we were little and we had muscular injuries we would go to the sobandera. *I don't know how to say that in English. Everyone knew who she was; she was like an . . . elder. What she did was physical and spiritual . . . it was in between a masseuse and a* curandera. *Perhaps something like a lay physical therapist? I don't know how to explain it. All I know is that it worked for us.*—Concha

An example of this was the traditional role of the *sobandera*. Latinas from south Texas to Colombia to Venezuela knew where to find the *sobandera*—the woman who fixed dislocated bones through therapeutic massage. It was a combination of healing the body and mind, plus a bit for the spirit. For some of us, we go for massage therapy to get similar results, and in some cases we are pleased to find that it is covered by our health insurance plan. But, on the whole, much of what is similar to "folk medicine" has been devalued by the mainstream medical community. As a result, some Latinas have been discouraged from seeking traditional medical care, at least until an illness has become very serious.

The good news for everyone is that mainstream medicine is beginning to accept and understand what Latinas have long known: there is a complex interrelationship between body, mind, and spirit.

MEDICAL APPROACHES BECOME LATINA FRIENDLY

ALTERNATIVE AND INTEGRATIVE APPROACHES, WHICH incorporate many aspects of folk medicine, have grown in use. According to the ongoing National Institutes of Health Study of Women's Health Across the Nation (SWAN), 43 percent of women used complementary and alternative medicine continuously, while 33 percent were sporadic users. The popularity of these methods clearly demonstrates the important role they play in our lives. While we may feel empowered when we use home-based and self-care approaches to our body, mind, and spirit, we also have to recognize the importance of contemporary diagnostics, medicines, and treatments.

> **HOT TEA IS GOOD AND CHICKEN SOUP IS BETTER.**
> Researchers at Cardiff University in Britain demonstrated that drinking a hot liquid, as opposed to one at room temperature, "provided immediate and sustained relief from symptoms of runny nose, cough, sneezing, sore throat, chilliness, and tiredness." *Caldo de pollo* (chicken soup) has been shown to have an additional substance that helps to clear your nose.

Happily, some alternative health care practices have even become part of the mainstream.

To make this blending of health care practices safe for us all, the National Center for Complementary and Alternative Medicine (NCCAM) was established in 1998. Part of the prestigious and scientifically rigorous National Institutes of Health, NCCAM oversees research on the diverse medical and health care systems, practices, and products that are not generally considered part of conventional, mainstream medicine. New centers for comprehensive or integrated health care are doing research to decipher the connections we Latinas have always recognized: our body, mind, and spirit are all part of who we are and what makes us thrive. And many other signs point to the type of health care system Latinas want.

We Latinas have always talked about health in more comprehensive ways. The source of our knowledge is the experiences we have and share with each other. Latinas are part of a community that knows health is intimate and personal.

UNDERSTANDING THE MEDICAL SYSTEM

I do not like going to see doctors. Whatever I need to do to take care of myself I will do. I have to take care of myself. —Female caller

IF STAYING HEALTHY IS THE GOAL, THEN SEEING A HEALTH CARE provider when we are well is essential to meeting that goal. Just as we know to take our children for "wellness visits," we also need to have those.

While one-third of Latinas do not have health insurance, even those of us who do have health insurance avoid going to see our health care providers. Too often our tendency is to wait until we are so sick that there are limits to which treatments will make us better.

For many of us—whether it is visiting a new health care provider, going for follow-up tests, or having to go to a hospital—encountering any aspect of the health care system feels like we are going into a different world. For most of us, this system is not part of our experience, we do not trust it, the people we meet are not always friendly, the path seems filled with obstacles, the language people use is not readily understandable, the food is not what we are used to, and we never know what we will encounter next. For Latinas to thrive, however, we must enter this system and use it for our own benefit.

It is easy to feel stranded or disoriented in this unfamiliar territory, yet we have to make so many decisions. People *within* the medical system talk about putting patients at the center of delivering health care, of being "patient centric," and of putting patients first. But while this may sound good, it may not always be as desirable as it seems. *Patient centric* suggests that the patient decides the best way to proceed. To some of us, it feels good to be in charge, but there are times when we do not want to be in charge and would like to be taken care of. Other times, we may be too tired, sick, conflicted, or overwhelmed to be in charge of navigating the way through the medical world.

Putting the patient in charge does not necessarily make health care experiences better for us. We feel on guard, and though most of us feel cared for by our individual health care provider, we do not have faith in the system as a whole. That is why health-related dissatisfaction among Latinas is pervasive. At the same time that we feel alienated, health care providers are frustrated by their inability to spend more time talking to us.

The need for a hospital visit or stay often magnifies all these fears and increases the level of distrust. Our care is often passed off from our familiar health care provider to a "hospitalist."

Hospitalist? You are probably wondering what or who that is. The hospitalist is the physician who coordinates your care with all the other medical staff while you are in the hospital. The problem is that it is unlikely that you have previously met the hospitalist. Additionally, the hospitalists change with each shift. Since our relationship with our health care provider is primary, the very organization of health care is incompatible with who we Latinas are and what we expect. We get asked the same questions many times by the different people who see us, and because the same questions get asked, we feel that no one was listening to us the last time we answered the same questions. We feel ignored and alone, and we wonder whether our care is being mishandled. This is not what is intended by any health care provider, though. No one went into the practice of medicine with the goal of providing substandard care.

The situation is complicated because at the same time that we are unhappy with the health care system, most practices, clinics, and hospitals are struggling to survive under the changing rules, economics, and ways of practicing medicine. There are new stresses for everyone involved. Does this mean that your visit to the health care provider will be negative and impersonal? Absolutely not. The intimacy you develop with your health care provider will frame the relationship.

But we also have to think in new ways. Neighborhood hospitals—more or less "full service" ones near our homes—are being replaced with more specialized regional facilities so that everyone can have access to the latest equipment and expert professionals. Also, some Latinas and their family members have been participating in the trend toward medical tourism, or travel outside of the United States for medical procedures. Staying "close to home" and in a familiar setting has less of a place in today's medicine. Keeping an open mind means understanding changes that may be coming soon, such as having a primary health care provider whom you visit with your cell phone.

Here are specific steps you can take to make your health care visits and exchanges with health care providers more productive.

CHECKLIST FOR VISITING YOUR HEALTH CARE PROVIDER:

1. Confirm your appointment and any special preparations you need to make (babysitter, not eating, transportation, translation, etc.).

2. Make a list of any questions you have.

3. Review your entries in the "About My Health" tools (in part 3).

4. Bring your "About My Health" entries so that you can be accurate about what you have been doing to stay healthy and what symptoms you are having.

5. If you have insurance, bring your insurance card.

6. If this is a first visit to a health care provider, get to the office early. You will need the time to carefully read and complete all the forms you are given to sign.

7. Answer all questions accurately.

8. Take notes or, if you prefer, bring someone with you to take notes. If you do not understand what you are being told, ask that it be explained to you again.

9. Make sure you understand when and how to take your medicines, what self-care steps you are to take, what the purpose was of any tests you had done, what alternatives to the recommendations might be helpful, and what the results from any tests or other procedures mean.

10. Ask when you should come back for a follow-up visit.

A NOTE ABOUT BEING INFORMED WHEN YOU GIVE CONSENT

In the United States you or someone representing you has to agree to treatment. This is known as *consent*. You give simple consent not only by what you say but also by what you do. You demonstrate consent when you follow the advice your health care provider gives you, including going for tests and buying your medicines.

My surgery was to take place in half an hour. I was naturally uneasy waiting in what, at best, was a holding room before the operation when a nurse walked in and gave me a clipboard with some forms to sign. I was already feeling disoriented, as hospitals are not my favorite place. As I skimmed over what I was about to sign, I asked, "What's this that I am agreeing to?" The nurse answered in a matter-of-fact tone, "Total abdominal hysterectomy." I was shocked as I said, "That's wrong. I am only supposed to have a cyst removed." The nurse looked at me in an annoyed way as she snapped, "This is what everyone signs—just in case more has to be done. Just sign it." At that point I refused to sign until I had spoken to my surgeon. —Jane Delgado

When situations are more likely to have bad outcomes— that is, they are riskier—your health care provider, the health care group or practice, or the hospital will ask you to give *informed consent*. Signing a form and giving informed consent mean that you understand what the risks are, what is going to be done, and what the expected outcomes are. Your informed consent must be given freely—that is, it must be voluntary—and this is especially true if you are going to be part of a research study. You cannot be coerced to participate.

It is your right and responsibility to be informed and to consent to the care you receive. That is why it is critical to carefully read any materials you are given to sign. Your health care provider will assume that you understand all that is said to you unless you state otherwise. It is much better to be clear in your communication, ask about what you do not understand, and repeat yourself, rather than to find that you have a body part missing or that your information is now shared with others.

> *I had my surgery because my doctor said it would help me have less painful periods. I don't know what he did, but now I can't have children. I hope to get married one day, but now I don't know if anyone will ever want to marry me.* —Female caller

At your first visit to a health care setting, you are usually given a lot of forms to sign. Most of us just sign them so we can get on with our appointment. This is not in your best interests. You need to carefully read all the forms that are given to you. The issue of consent is an essential part of your health care.

When being admitted to some hospitals, you may be asked to sign forms stating that any health care provider can treat you and that medical students can participate in your care. For surgery, your health care provider sometimes will give you the forms for informed consent beforehand, so that you can read them at home and bring the completed forms to the hospital. Do not sign them until all your questions have been answered. If you are not clear about what such statements mean, you need to find someone who can talk to you about the forms and explain what specific statements mean. If what you are told is not acceptable to you, then you have the right to refuse. At that point, you and your health care provider will have to decide on other arrangements.

One thing's for certain: today's health care system is not your mother's *medicina* (medicine)—and for that we are all grateful. Mainstream medicine now includes aspects of alternative and folk medicines, science holds much promise, and the health care system continues to evolve.

For Latinas, we have to recognize the obvious: the health care system can feel disorienting and even hostile. Our challenge is to do what we, as Latinas, do best: find our own path through the health care system.

IT WILL GET BETTER: ADVANCES IN SCIENCE

BEING ACTIVE IN OUR HEALTH CARE HAS A REAL IMPACT ON our lives. Even bigger health benefits are around the corner, especially if we maintain and enhance our health. Medical science is on the threshold of discoveries that will make our health care better and more relevant to us.

Too many Latinas have been discouraged from having any enthusiasm about science. It is through scientific discoveries, however, that exciting possibilities are being developed that could radically affect your lives—and your children's lives. The problem is, it takes ten to fifteen years for what is learned in the laboratory to be applied to actual patient care—and even longer for that knowledge to reach Latinas. What makes progress even more complicated and confusing for everyone is the fact that new developments sometimes overturn views about what is right and that they often require a rethinking of assumptions and practices. Progress is not always a straight line; sometimes you have to loop back and take a different path to go in the right direction.

A good place to begin talking about the future is to share what I have learned about three especially promising areas of research and development: the human genome, nanotechnology, and human regeneration. These may sound very futuristic, but they are realities in the making today.

THE HUMAN GENOME

Amazingly, the differences in the genes from one person to another are less than 3 percent. We are more alike than we ever imagined. Obviously, small differences can make a tremendous difference.

Every species has one genome—that is, a set of instructions given to cells so they will form one new member of that particular species. For humans, our genome is made up of approximately twenty-three thousand genes. Our genes provide the instructions so that each person develops from one cell into an organism with seventy-five trillion to a hundred trillion cells. There are some powerful messages for Latinas in our genetic code that will improve our health.

WHAT DO YOU WANT TO KNOW?
As you think about your health, you have to start thinking about how much information you want. While in 2008 the cost for determining a person's complete genetic blueprint was $100,000, some companies are working to reduce the cost to $5,000 and eventually $1,000 and even less than that.

The questions that each Latina has to ask herself are, How much information do I really want to have? What do I do with all that information? Will I use the information to change how I live? Would I prefer not to know that I'm at risk for certain diseases?

When scientists started to study and map the human genome, they believed they would be able to identify which gene is responsible for each disease, and even which genes determine our behavior. The hope was that with this information it would be possible to figure out which diseases a person would be most likely to get, as well as explain why some people are more likely than others to "bounce back" from difficult life events. The assumption was that if you knew there was a gene for a specific disease or trait and you had that gene, then you could be fairly certain you would get that disease or exhibit that behavior.

> At one point scientists thought they knew a lot because they had mapped the human genome. Then in 2008 Dr. J. Craig Venter, pioneer and leading scientist in the world of genomic research, and his team showed the scientific community that there was more work to be done, as both sides of the DNA in a gene were not identical. It seemed that scientists had mapped only half of the human genome.

Many people anticipated that the early human genome research would lead to "gene therapy" to treat or prevent diseases. They also thought the research findings would provide a way of explaining why there were variations in how we respond to life events. As it turns out, this type of thinking grossly distorted our understanding of disease and behavior. A good example is diabetes in the Hispanic community.

In the new millennium Hispanics were bombarded with news about the diabetes epidemic and how Hispanics were more likely to get the disease. Since Latinas heard so often that diabetes was epidemic in our families and communities, many assumed it was in our genes. In a burst of *fatalismo* (fatalism), some Latinas resigned themselves to the fact that they would get diabetes. They believed that being Hispanic meant there was nothing they could do to avoid getting diabetes.

Today we know that the case for diabetes in the Hispanic community was not well stated. There is no single gene for diabetes, and diabetes in the Hispanic community may be due to a variety of reasons. Moreover, what researchers are discovering is that *diabetes* may be a name that includes many diseases.

As scientists learned more about the human genome, they discovered that, in the end, exercise, diet, and weight may matter far more than genes. For the overwhelming majority of diseases there is no single causative gene or set of genes. The exceptions are in those rare diseases that are caused by a genetic disorder, such as Huntington's disease.

In most cases, however, our genes only increase the likelihood of some characteristic or disease occurring. They do not ensure that we will have it. Instead, recent research has focused on the question of what turns a gene—or more likely, a set of genes—on or off. It seems that our experiences, exposures, and even our emotions may turn genes on or off. In other words, whatever determines whether we have a disease or a characteristic is not dictated by our genes alone but is also encouraged or muffled by the world around us. *Cultura* and *familia* are important. Equally important is the fact that each person is unique in how the various influences come together and affect health. What works best often differs from person to person.

JUST-FOR-YOU MEDICINES
By unraveling the complexity of the human genome, researchers are developing new treatments that are tailored to the individual (pharmacogenomics). The future of medicine will be in the development of treatments specific to the illnesses of each person. This will maximize positive outcomes and minimize negative side effects. The one-size-fits-all approach to medicine will be the past; precision medicine is the future.

Epigenomics

The field of epigenomics—the study of what makes a good gene stay on and what must be done to turn off a bad gene—was born out of the need to understand the levers that activate disease and wellness. "Epigenomics will build upon

I know about genes, but what do you mean epigenomics? *How do you spell it? I never heard of it? I thought it was all in your genes.*—Carmen

our new knowledge of the human genome and help us better understand the role of the environment in regulating genes that protect our health or make us more susceptible to disease," predicted Dr. Elias A. Zerhouni in 2008, when he was the director of the National Institutes of Health.

Fortunately, the full account of this mystery is being written even now. The promise in this area is enormous, and as Latinas, we have to stay aware of how these discoveries are changing medicine.

NANOMEDICINE

Another area where medicine is changing has to do with the use of some very, very tiny materials. *Nano* comes from *nanometer*, which is one billionth of a meter. In recent years, researchers have produced molecules, robots, and machines that are invisible to the naked eye and to most microscopes. Each nanochemical, nanorobot, or nanomachine is 100 nanometers or less in size. In other words, the dot above this *i* could hold thousands of these nanosubstances. Substances or objects this small can be programmed to go into a living cell and change the way it operates.

Nanomedicine is the use of nanotechnology or nanochemicals to improve our health. According to the Food and Drug Administration (FDA), nanoscale materials are being used in medical devices, prescription drugs, over-the-counter (OTC) drugs like sunscreens, food and color additives, dietary supplements, and cosmetics. There is even the promise of surgery without having to cut through flesh. The concern at this point is that the FDA has not set standards for labeling, measuring, or detecting these materials. At the same time, this technology is already on a very fast track, and its use is spreading. In March 2006 there were 212 nanotechnology-based products; by August 2008 there were 803. It may not make the evening news, but every day we are exposed to these unregulated substances at an increasing rate.

CANCER AND NANOMEDICINE

The hope is that nanorobots and nanocompounds will target specific molecules without damaging healthy molecules. This approach would help in early diagnosis, targeted treatment, and even prevention of cancer.

The question for Latinas is, Will these minuscule particles affect *us* in unique ways?

We already know that Latinas and non-Hispanic whites often metabolize medicines differently. How will the new nanomolecules change our health? Early indications are that there is reason for concern. There are documented findings that inhaled nanoparticles get lodged in the lungs and are toxic in the same way as asbestos—a disturbing fact. As we move forward with nanotechnologies, Latinas need to be aware of the potential benefits and risks that exist.

We need to keep alert with respect to all things nano.

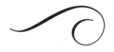

REGENERATION: GROWING YOUR OWN

Juan Enriquez, the brilliant author of *As the Future Catches You—How Genomics and Other Forces Are Changing Your Life, Work, Health and Wealth,* makes it clear that cells—human or otherwise—take instruction. For instance, with the right set of genetic instructions, a seed will produce an orange. But if the instruction set is incorrect or changed, what grows will not be an orange but perhaps a lemon, a grapefruit, or a tangerine.

Given what we know about the human genome and nanotechnology, we are now starting to understand how to give cells new instructions—that is, to reprogram cells. The new instructions at the cellular level can help us heal parts of our bodies that are damaged, or they can prevent further damage from occurring. This entire area of medical science, known as regeneration, is relatively new, and discoveries are being made each day.

Here are a few examples of recent breakthroughs. First, with our teeth. Scientists at the NIH have learned how to grow new teeth by giving certain instructions to adult stem cells found in the material near wisdom teeth. Next, with our hearts. In 2007 the NIH hosted a scientific symposium on cardiovascular regenerative medicine. The goal was to better understand cells that naturally reside in the heart, growth factors to stimulate formation of new blood vessels (vascular regeneration) and to repair or regenerate cardiac tissue (cardiac regeneration), and technologies for monitoring cell activity. With more being learned each day about such possibilities, we all stand to benefit in major ways that will help us live longer and better.

MEDICINE TAILORED TO THE INDIVIDUAL

All these advances and others like them will lead to a practice of medicine that is tailored to the individual. Just as we know from clothes shopping that one size does not fit all, scientists are discovering that the success of a treatment is sometimes due to differences at the cellular level, and they know that certain treatments will be successful because of the makeup of an individual cell. Researchers are working hard to deliver the right medicine at the right time to the right individual. But this is proving very challenging. For now, we, as Latinas, must try to maintain ourselves in the best possible condition so that, as these breakthroughs become part of health care, we will be able to make good use of them. Much change is coming to our health care through the promises of science and the new health care systems that address our integrated sense of our health. The path to even better health care for Latinas is right in front of us.

Caring for Ourselves: Body, Mind, and Spirit

YES, IT IS TRUE: OUR BODY, MIND, AND SPIRIT ARE INTEGRATED. Scientists have found that there are special connections that link genes, the brain, and social behavior. Specifically, what happens in our life in terms of environment, stress, nutrition, and a host of other factors can change gene expression. We may not be able to see this process or control it, but it does happen.

> Serotonin is a chemical in the brain that plays a big role in depression and also seems to also have a role with respect to how our immune system functions. The brain communicates with the immune system. That is one way our bodies respond to what we feel. That is why stress is not something we should just manage; we need to reduce it.
> (Plus stress gives women more of that dangerous belly fat.)
>   Although stress causes our bodies to respond in a variety of ways, research consistently finds that stress is also accompanied by chronic inflammation. The result is that our immune systems do not function as well as they could—or should. Dr. Janice Kiecolt-Glaser, of the Ohio State University College of Medicine, conducted research and stated that based on her research, "Stress made 55-year-olds have 90-year-old immune systems."

Basic to good health is being able to listen to the messages that we get from our bodies and to recognize the impact that our feelings have on our health. This will be easier for some of us than for others. I do believe that as Latinas we are often better listeners to our bodies and our inner selves because we are more aware and accepting of the connection between body, mind, and spirit. Perhaps this ability has to do with the way we can say things in Spanish, or maybe it is just that emotional expression is an accepted part of our lives and part of who we are.

Understanding that our body, mind, and spirit work together can enhance our health and our ability to get well and stay well. When we see our health as the result of healthy habits—regular medical care, good eating habits, loving relationships, joyful sexuality, meaningful fulfillment of our emotional and spiritual needs—we have the greatest chance for happiness and wellness. Too often the health messages that are sent to all women are lost on us because we do not see how those apply to our lives. We hear the messages, but they have no impact on us because they don't seem to reflect what is relevant to us, as Latinas. I decided to take the key messages I believe are essential for us and change them according to the experiences and values that Latinas have shared with me wherever I have gone.

These are hugely important steps to make a part of your life.

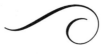

AVOIDING ALL SMOKE

MOST LATINAS SHRUG OFF WARNINGS NOT TO SMOKE because they do not smoke. But young Latinas are smoking more. Latinas of all ages need to focus on the broader message about smoking: Not only should you not smoke (firsthand smoke), but you also need to stay away from places where people smoke (secondhand smoke) or where there is smoke. This includes the barbecue pit, despite that nice cooking smell. Then there is the matter of that nasty smell that hovers when a smoker walks by or that gets into your clothes and hair because you have been near a smoker. That is now called thirdhand smoke, and it is dangerous, too. Smoke—first-, second-, or thirdhand is simply not good for your lungs.

When your lungs do not work well, your heart does not work well either. The dangers of being around a smoker are especially bad for Latinas who are pregnant. If you have any doubt about how unappealing smoking is, think about the old saying "Kissing a smoker is like licking an ashtray." It may be graphic, but it's also true.

And be certain about this: if you do smoke, now is an excellent time to quit.

GOING FOR ANNUAL WELLNESS VISITS

You know, I really never focused on my health much. There are so many other things that I have to do. I exercise and I eat well and that's enough for me. I'm fine.—Female caller

ALL LATINAS NEED TO ESTABLISH A PLACE WHERE THEY WILL go for regular, ongoing health care. There are programs to help us, regardless of our resources. Too often we Latinas tend to see a health care provider only when we are sick, but many illnesses are most treatable in their early stages when we may not feel very sick. We need to see our health care provider so that we will be treated early and can avoid complications. For example, some Latinas with untreated chlamydia will end up unable to have children. Regular Pap tests are especially important for Latinas, who have a greater risk for cervical cancer. Diabetes that is not controlled can lead to blindness or the need to amputate a foot. Be alert to the fact that often the person who has a sexually transmitted disease (STD) has no symptoms. Latinas with more than one intimate partner should get screened for chlamydia and gonorrhea. This is especially true for Latinas younger than twenty-five, as they are more likely to get these diseases. (In Part Two, we look at these and other specific conditions among Latinas.)

Ignoring a symptom will not make the disease go away; the earlier we identify a problem, the more likely it is that treatment will be successful. Wellness is the goal, and seeing a health care provider on a regular basis is key.

Eating Good and Good-for-You Foods

_____

Focusing on foods that keep you feeling good and help you stay in shape is a key part of healthiness. When you set goals for good eating, you are also taking care of your overall well-being and self-esteem, especially regarding what weight is best for your health. For Latinas and most other women the term *obesity* is offensive. The worst part is that having a "Reduce Obesity" campaign turns off the very people that the well-intended health message is supposed to reach. The area of obesity is a prime example of when there is a mismatch between the Latina experience and what we are told.

We like ourselves. This was the conclusion of the 2004 *Dove Report: Challenging Beauty.* It documented some important differences between Latinas and other women. Latinas were more likely to say that their "looks" were above average and that their beauty was above average. Latinas were also more likely to "like how they look" and more likely to say that they were "looking beautiful." Positive self-esteem is very important to health.

If you are not feeling all that positive, though, forget about trying to achieve some goal of perfection. None of us is perfect or will achieve a "perfect" body. Even those Latinas we think of as gorgeous are not perfect. Whatever images you are seeing on the TV screen or in magazines that make Latina stars seem perfect come from working at creating those images—and from plenty of professional touching up. For these women, looking as if they were perfect is part of their job.

For certain, there are bumps where you may wish there were none, and your skin may not be the way you want it to be. That is all okay because those imperfections are what make you unique. What is attractive is always in the eye of the beholder, and that changes, based on all sorts of situations.

> In 2006, after a fashion model died of anorexia, Spain became the first country to say no to overly thin models. As the Spanish regional official in Madrid, Concha Guerra, said, "Fashion is a mirror and many teenagers imitate what they see on the catwalk." (In 2009 Guerra became vice-minister of culture and tourism for Spain.)

Given these facts, we have to learn to love ourselves—and that includes the aspects we may want to improve. You are you. To be healthy, you have to appreciate the body you have. Loving your body means that taking care of it is at the top of the wellness list for every Latina.

So where does that leave us? The "instant health" look that comes with makeup and blush is meaningless. For many of us, being *gordita* (pleasantly plump) is what we see and value. For Hispanics, a woman can never be too rich, but she can be too thin. We also know of family members and friends who lived long lives even though they had some excess weight. The issue is to decide what is right for us.

Beginning in the 1990s the government recognized that people in the United States were getting heavier. Since being heavier was correlated with the full gamut of chronic health problems (heart disease, diabetes, hypertension, and so on), the strategy was too reduce the chronic health problems by vigorously attacking obesity. Government, foundations, and industries began to tell us that we were fat and that being fat was awful. At the same time, science was telling us that the relationship between weight and some health problems was more complex than had been imagined.

Nevertheless, our understanding of the role of excess weight became even more complex as more comparative data became available about the measure of the relationship between weight and height known as the body mass index (BMI). The research showed that people who were overweight (BMI of 25.0 to 29.9) had better health outcomes than people who were normal (BMI 20.0 to 25.0) or underweight. Moreover, the greatest health risks were for those people who were severely obese (BMI 35.0 to 39.9), morbidly obese (BMI 40.0 to 49.0), or superobese (BMI over 50.0). Even with this knowledge, we Latinas were continuing to be told our BMIs were too high, our waists too big, or our weight too much—or, sometimes, all three at once. The messages turned out to be more stigmatizing than inspiring.

There was no need for an expensive study to document what we all know. Looking at ourselves, our families, and our friends, we can see when we are carrying excess weight. And while we may want a few extra pounds to soften us, we know that too much extra weight is not good.

It turns out, however, that all fat is not the same. We have brown fat, which is good and burns energy, and white fat, which is for storage and accumulates around our organs when we have excess amounts. The white fat is the dangerous kind. Both types of fat are critical to a well-functioning endocrine system. (So don't even think about liposuction, as it eliminates the "good" fat as well as the "bad" that you need to be healthy and be fit.)

To complicate matters, we also know how changes in our hormones affect our proportions. With the onset of menopause we have less estrogen and the fat migrates elsewhere. The good news is that it migrates away from our hips and our hips get smaller. The bad news is that it goes to our belly area, which is a dangerous area to have excess fat. That is why we have to change how much we eat as we get older, since our body needs less food to function well. If we continue eating just as we did when younger, our belly will get larger and larger. To make matters worse, when we women are under stress, our body produces more cortisol, a substance that increases fat storage in the belly. The only good news here is that while our belly may be larger, this is the area that is most responsive to healthy eating and increased physical activity.

The truth is, even though each of us wants to be healthy and look good, all of the recent years' dire messages about what's wrong with us have not encouraged enough of us to take the necessary steps. A 2009 analysis of the healthy lifestyles habits in adults compared those for U.S. women in 1988 through 1994 to those for women in 2001 through 2006. In these studies women were actually weighed, and the results showed that the percentage of Hispanic women with a high BMI stayed relatively stable while the percentage increased for non-Hispanic white women and for African American women. The numbers only support what both Hispanic and non-Hispanic women have told me: some of us were tired of being told that another thing was wrong with us, others took the negative messages as another example of how we were "less than," and many of us just gave up after many attempts at losing weight.

THE SHIFTING NATURE OF BODY MASS INDEX (BMI)

In 1998, the NIH brought U.S. definitions into line with World Health Organization (WHO) guidelines, lowering the normal weight cutoff from BMI 27 to BMI 25. This made approximately thirty million Americans, previously "technically healthy" to "technically overweight." WHO also recommended lowering the normal/overweight threshold for Southeast Asian body types to around BMI 23. Further revisions will emerge from clinical studies of different body types. Already the data indicate that for African Americans the thresholds should be raised. We are still waiting for findings that apply to Latinas.

Dr. Jules Hirsch, a research physician at Rockefeller University, conducted research for more than fifty years to find out why some people were fat. He concluded that 70 percent of the differences in weight between people were due to the genes inherited from their parents, as opposed to bad habits they had learned from their parents. Extensive research with twins who had been separated and children who had been adopted documented that the family gene pool had an enormous impact on individuals. Dr. Hirsch's data also documented why it was so difficult for people to maintain their healthy weight after having lost excess weight. Nevertheless, the findings were controversial. Finally, in 2007, *Science* reported that a specific variation in a particular gene (designated FTO) had a major impact on the size of people's bodies. People with two copies of this variation carried eight more pounds than people who lacked that gene. This conclusion was based on data from thirty-nine thousand people.

What this means is that maintaining a healthy weight is harder work for some of us than it is for others. This is another reason why you should work with your health care provider to determine what is a reasonable plan for you to follow.

Obviously, there are entire industries that depend on convincing you that you will lose (or gain) weight if you try their product or method or idea. But as you know, their claims are

I have always weighed a lot, and for just as long I have felt uncomfortable about it. My best friend Lucy was just the opposite of that; she was very comfortable with her size. She knew she was full figured and was honest about liking to eat. One time when we were going out to dinner together, the host was leading us to a very nice table for two. It makes me laugh at the joyfulness with which Lucy politely said, "Oh no thank you... we need a big table. I am very hungry and we are going to need eat a lot of space for all the food we are going to eat!"—Alicia

No matter how little I eat, I always seem to gain weight.—Elena

When he called me, I got so nervous. There was a box of chocolate truffles nearby, and before I knew it I had eaten the entire box. I guess I don't even realize what or how much I eat when I am nervous.— Lianne

When I am depressed, I just cannot eat. It makes the food get stuck in my mouth. I cannot either chew or swallow. My throat is so choked up that the food will not go down. Food is the last thing that is on my mind when I am depressed. —Nadia

Get nutrients from food. Whole foods are better than
dietary supplements. —Marian L. Neuhouser,
Fred Hutchinson Cancer Research Center, Seattle, WA

focused on selling their product. The fact is that your body can be healthier if you are patient and consistently work to stay fit for the rest of your life. Healthy eating and regular exercise must be part of your daily life.

As Latinas, we know that in our community and in many other communities it is more appealing for women to be curvier and rounder. The issue is to find the shape and size at which you are both comfortable and fit. The best goal is not to achieve a certain number but instead to be as fit as possible and to maintain a healthy range for your body.

For many of us, food is one of the connections that tie us to our families and community. We eat the way we do to nourish our bodies and experience pleasure. Food delights our senses; that's why we have taste buds. The challenge is to think about eating in a way that nourishes us, is satisfying, and helps us maintain a healthy weight. If food were only about nourishment, then we could eat a powdered product that had all the nutrients we needed.

The most important challenge is deciding what is good for you. The secret to healthy eating is to think about what you are going to eat. Here are some ways we can nourish our Latina bodies well.

1. **AVOID EXCESS.** Food is the fuel for your body, and you have to eat enough to provide fuel for your daily activities. This means that you are supposed to eat to be healthy, not to be stuffed. Rushing meals will cause you to overeat because it takes a while (about twenty minutes) for your brain to recognize that you are full. There are several things you can do to slow down your eating:

    - *Eat smaller bites and eat more slowly.*
    - *Serve yourself in courses. This slows down the sequence of eating.*
    - *Engage in more conversation, since your mouth is empty when you are speaking.*
    - *Put your fork down between bites.*
    - *As you get older, you will feel full after eating less food.*
    - *As you reduce your level of physical activity, you will need less fuel for your body.*

2. **EAT FOR NOURISHMENT.** Eating because you are anxious or sad or happy is not the purpose of food. Whatever your emotional needs are, food is not what you need to resolve them. Be honest with yourself about what makes you eat.

3. **KNOW WHAT YOU ARE EATING.** Be informed and read food labels, which are there to make you aware of what is in the food you're eating. Some of us just look at the calories in products, but you also need to focus on how many servings

there are in a container and how much saturated fat, trans fat (which should be 0, zero!), cholesterol, sodium, carbohydrates, and other such things are in the food. The serving size indicated on labels is what I often find amusing. Recently, I bought some frozen plantains. The label said there were four servings in the container, but there were only three pieces of plantain—very confusing.

The nutritional value is not the same for all products, no matter how similar they may be to each other. Whole wheat pasta is a good example. There are many brands of whole wheat pasta. The amount of carbohydrates in a two-ounce serving can range from twenty-nine grams to forty-two grams, depending on the company's ingredients and manufacturing processes.

4. **AVOID THE WHITE STUFF: SUGAR, WHITE FLOUR, WHITE RICE, WHITE POTATOES, SALT (SODIUM), LARD, AND FAT.** Many of us know to avoid white sugar, but it is also good to avoid foods that our bodies quickly change into sugar. Such foods would be cookies, cakes, breads, and other foods made from white flour, as well as white rice and white potatoes. For the same reason, orange juice, apple juice, and some fruits also should be avoided. You can reduce the sodium you eat by reading the food labels and choosing products that have less. Canned tomato juices, for instance, have widely varying amounts of sodium because of differences in the manufacturers' recipes. Regardless of the color of the salt or its place of origin, avoiding it is best. Our bodies need very little sodium to function.

Lard and the fat in meat should be avoided because they are not good for our circulatory system. The reasons are many and well documented. Recently, however, the

Minnesota Department of Health reaffirmed another reason to avoid fat: "Dietary intake of animal fat is the major route of exposure [to dioxins—a group of related compounds that have negative health effects] for the general population. For most people, eating a varied, balanced, low-fat diet will result in reduced fat intake and will reduce exposure to dioxins. A low-fat diet, aside from reducing your exposure to dioxins, also will reduce your chances of developing heart disease, high blood pressure, certain cancers, and diabetes."

5. **ENJOY IN MODERATION THE BROWN STUFF,** which includes foods made from whole wheat or unprocessed wheat, whole grains, beans, unrefined sugar, and nuts. Our bodies change these carbohydrates into sugar slowly, and they are rich in fiber. You still have to be careful about how much you eat and the number of calories.

6. **GOOD CHOICES ARE RED, ORANGE, BLUE, AND GREEN.** Tomatoes, carrots, blueberries, and all salad leaves and vegetables that are green bring lots of tasty and good nutrients into your body. These are rich in many of the vitamins and minerals we need.

7. **THINK ABOUT THE FAT AND OILS.** Lean cuts of chicken, pork, beef, and lamb can all be part of healthy eating. Just be sure to trim off the fat and eat smaller portions. Olive oil and canola oil are good in moderation, and a little bit of butter for flavoring is okay. Remember, you should have no trans fats.

8 **EAT AT HOME.** Eating at home is a good way to be in better control of what you eat. It also saves money and if you plan it right it will save you time.

It is hard to make healthy choices, but those are the ones that will bring us the best results. As we make healthier choices about what we eat, there will be changes in our bodies, too. While we may like the way we look at a given shape and size, the main goal is to be as healthy as possible. One Latina told me that the greatest benefit from getting to be a size 14 was that she no longer experienced knee pain. That had not been her goal, but it turned out to be a terrific outcome.

GETTING FIT FOR YOUR HEART, FLEXIBILITY, AND STRENGTH

LATINAS ARE THE WOMEN LEAST LIKELY TO EXERCISE. Perhaps it is because our work and our families are more likely to leave us physically exhausted. When we have free time, we just want to sit and do nothing. But in order to fully enjoy our lives, we need to make movement part of the way we relax. There are ways to move that can be fun and good for us. Take dancing, which is good for our heart and flexibility. We can then consider adding something to increase our strength. The goal is for each Latina to be able to move freely and remain independent for as long as possible.

When I am in school, I know that I should exercise but I do not seem to have the time. I know that it makes me feel better, but I still do not seem to do it. Next semester I will work on doing more exercise. —Isabel

I don't have the money to join a gym.—Consuelo

I am too tired when I get home from work.—Radio caller

Why do we all agree that movement is important for our health yet still do not do enough? Perhaps it is because Latinas did not go to schools where physical activity was part of the curriculum. For Latinas with one parent born outside the United States, only 43 percent participated in organized or team sports while growing up. For nonimmigrant girls the participation rate was 65 percent, and for nonimmigrant boys it was 72 percent. It could also be that the competitive nature of team sports was not appealing; we Latinas play for the camaraderie and for fun. Or maybe we were traumatized at a young age because we were not picked to be on a team.

Regardless of what shadows from the past exist or what obstacles there are in the present, we have to figure out a way to increase our physical activity to healthier levels. The benefits of movement to our body are many. Aerobic activity is good for our heart; strengthening is good for our muscles, bones, and joints; and flexibility is good for our muscles. There is growing evidence that regular exercise increases our ability to engage in higher-level thinking and helps keep depression and anxiety at bay. Many researchers are trying to understand all the complex ways that exercise contributes to our brain biochemistry and seems to alleviate symptoms of depression.

Given all the positive outcomes from physical activity, the challenge remains to incorporate it in our lives. There are a variety of strategies that work. You just have to try some and see which one works for you. At different points in your life you may need to shift strategies. What motivates you when you are twenty-five will not be what keeps you working to be fit at sixty-five.

MAKE A PLAN TO SUIT YOUR LIFE

The first step in getting fit is to be realistic about your goals. You have to know the limitations of what you can do and how much you can do. To make a plan that will work for you, consider the following steps.

Getting Started.

Make sure you check with your health care provider to determine what is best for you. Start as soon as you can. It is never too late to start. Even someone in her fifties, sixties, or seventies will see significant health benefits.

Commitment.

Madonna and Gwyneth Paltrow put in at least two hours a day, six days a week with a personal trainer because how they look is essential to their business. You have to commit to being fit because it is essential to your health and overall quality of life.

You also have to be realistic about how your body will change. Your posture may improve, but you will not grow taller. Your stomach may get strong, but you may not end up with a flat stomach. What will happen with regular physical activity is that your heart will work better, it will be easier for you to lift items, and you will be able to move better. We also know that your mood will improve. Whatever your goal is, it has to be realistic for you, your physical condition, and your circumstances.

While at an earlier stage in your life you may have been able to dance, run, and play sports, as your responsibilities increase you will have to make choices as to which activities are reasonable for you. It may be that walking in place during commercials is your first step away from being a couch potato.

Time.

Given that you are very busy, making time for exercise will take effort on your part. The more you make physical activity part of your daily life, the more energy you will have. The time you put into being fit is an incredible investment because the returns you get will benefit every aspect of your life.

If you are just beginning a program at home, you need to look at your week and see where you can carve out thirty minutes at least three times a week. When beginning, you may use only ten minutes per day, but you need to get into the habit of setting aside time for yourself. If your plate is full, then this is a good time to ask others for help.

Activities.

A ten-minute stroll after you finish eating is a good place to start. In many countries that is the custom, and it is one that offers a lot of good outcomes. As we rely more on cars, this healthy activity has been erased from our daily routine. Walking is the best exercise you can do because you can do it for the rest of your life. All you need is a comfortable pair of shoes.

If you have access to a pool, swimming is particularly good for people with excess weight or those who have joint problems. Physical activity should not cause pain or discomfort. "Feeling the burn" may mean that you are injuring yourself. Ligaments and tendons that may have shortened and tightened later in life become lower back pains and foot pain (plantar fasciitis). The goal is to move your muscles. Muscle health is about using your muscles, not building bulk. As you know, bulk is a function of genes and gender. You may also want to look at local community-based organizations that offer classes you may enjoy. At different times of the year you may decide to pursue different interests. The important thing is to keep moving.

Getting Support.
There are many ways to get support for your exercise. Some people stay motivated if they enroll in a class, and others need to exercise with a friend. Some make exercise part of an ongoing family activity. Others prefer to use the time they do their physical activity as a period for quiet reflection and nothing else. There is no one way that is best. Just find the one that works for you. Sometimes just keeping a log of what you have done is sufficient to motivate you to keep going. If one type of support does not work, try another.

Staying on the Program.
If you go off your program, you can always get back on. We all know how difficult it is to stay on track, but we have to be honest and know what will work for us. Think about physical activity as you do about brushing your teeth—as something you have to do every day. You can skip a day, but you must make it a part of your daily life. And while you can get a set of dentures if you have totally neglected your teeth, you cannot get a new body.

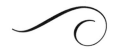

Sleeping Soundly and Sufficiently

It seems that we, as Latinas, fall into the groups that are particularly at risk for sleep deprivation, such as parents, teenagers, and shift workers. But to nourish and replenish ourselves, we need to get enough sleep. This is sometimes difficult because our responsibilities may make it difficult to have a regular schedule. At other times we may not have enough hours to do all the things we need to do and, as a solution, decide to sacrifice our sleeping time. While we can do this on occasion, we cannot do this too often. If we do, we end up damaging our body. Additionally, when we lack sufficient sleep, we do not make good decisions, we become irritable, and we are likely to have memory problems. But the fact that we take the need for sleep for granted is not surprising.

Only recently did the Centers for Disease Control and Prevention (CDC) begin considering sleep and sleep disorders as public health challenges. For a long time sleep was considered a passive activity that didn't mean very much to our overall health. Research has documented, however, that lack of sleep is associated with diabetes, depression, heart disease, and immune system problems. For example, less sleep results in less resistance to colds. Ironically, we still are not certain why we sleep. Although there are many theories, none has been shown to be definitive.

What is certain is that sleeping, like eating, is something we must do to live. There is no exact formula to tell you how much sleep you need each day, but research has shown that the best range for adults is six to nine hours. You need to figure out how much time you need to sleep so you can be alert most of the day. This is something you figure out through trial and error and is particularly difficult for people who work shifts, especially when those shifts change. Keeping track in your health journal should help you decipher how much sleep is best for you. Once you know what you need then you have to work to make sure that you get the sleep you need. Your body depends on it.

ENJOYING SEXUAL INTIMACY

> *María approached me to tell me about her mother. In the 1930s María's mother had married a younger man. At that time, those types of liaisons were considered scandalous at best. Nevertheless, María knew that she had benefited from the age difference between her parents. They had a happy life. She explained that although her mother had died when María was relatively young, she had at least been left with a father to take care of her.*
>
> *Then María told me about her own life. She had fallen in love and married a man who was twelve years older than she. As she looked down, you could see the sadness as she added, "I still love my husband, but we are more like a brother and sister. That's okay because he is a good husband."*
>
> *I didn't know what to say, as the resignation in her voice was as clear as the pain her words communicated. And then María looked up at me with a hopeful smile and said, "My friends who are widows and dating... I tell those friends of mine to marry a younger man. It's better that way."*

YES, MARÍA, SEXUAL INTIMACY IS IMPORTANT FOR US AT ALL ages because it is one way we care for ourselves and show how we care for the person we love. The data only support what we know: Latinas enjoy sexual intimacy.

But sometimes social pressures make us engage in activities that do not give us the full benefits. For example, "hooking up," or having casual sexual relationships, is only about the mechanics. Too often when Latinas allow themselves to think about their last sexual partner, they are left with a "Now what?" type of feeling. The sexual tension was reduced, but that was all that happened. The process of sexual intimacy is more of an evolving journey.

Our relationships are intense, and sexual intimacy is an important way to express the closeness we are sharing. The physical aspects should be about mutual joy and pleasure. Sexual sharing should be playful and fun, and it should be something you willingly do. Coercion of any kind—from the subtlety of words to the use of physical force—is not acceptable. Sexual intimacy based on coercion is a violation of you, as a woman.

You must feel comfortable talking to your partner about what you like and do not like. If you feel that you cannot talk to your partner or that this person does not listen or value what you say, then you should seriously reconsider whether physical intimacy should be included as part of the relationship. Sexual intimacy between two people who love each other can be a form of nourishment. You must be honest with yourself about your relationships.

We Latinas today are neither the feminists of the 1960s nor the vision of independent women in the twenty-first century that those feminists thought that we would be. Latinas of every age feel pulled in different directions and confused by the culture's pervasive sexual messages. During the sixties, coming to terms with our own sexuality was supposed to liberate and free women to pick our partners. The intent was for us to be free to choose our partners, instead of having to wait to be "picked." Instead, the expectation has become for women to be sexually available for men, with insufficient focus on what women want.

It is obvious that over the past fifty years some things have not changed. Young women are still pressured to be sexually active. Other women adhere to the practice of friends with benefits because it is less complicated and easier to manage. For still others, oral sex is not considered either intimate or sex, just an expectation that needs to be met. And many health problems related to sex remain. For instance, the data on HIV and sexually transmitted diseases (STDs) remind us that Latinas desperately need to practice what we know about safer sex—we need to use condoms.

We need to remember that men who have sex with men and women are more likely to use a condom when they are with another man. We don't know why this is the case, but it is likely that the women are less demanding about the use of the condom. This is consistent with data showing that Latinas are the women whose partners are least likely to use a condom. A condom will protect you from most STDs. Talking to your partner about their other partners is critical to your own well-being. (We look at these issues more in Part Two.) Suffice it to say that we still have a lot to learn about taking care of ourselves while also celebrating our own pleasure and nurturing our desire for physical intimacy. What we do already understand is that for sexual intimacy to be nourishing, we need to value ourselves and our relationships. Sexual intimacy is more than satisfying the body; it is about fulfilling our emotional desires and needs, too.

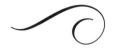

PROMOTING CLEAN AIR AND SAFE WATER

Sometimes I have trouble breathing. Do you really think it could be the environment?—Monica

FOR DECADES THOSE OF US WHO LIVE IN THE UNITED STATES assumed we had clean air and safe drinking water. Recent news coverage has made it clear that these assumptions are no longer true. Contamination of our air and water continues to increase. Moreover, we know that there are serious health consequences from our exposure to even minute amounts of contaminated or hazardous substances. To take care of ourselves, we need to be aware of the environmental factors compromising our lives and know what steps we can take to reduce the bad effects.

CLEAN OUTDOOR AIR

Latinas need to be very concerned about air quality, because we are very likely to live in a community where the air quality is compromised. It is also well documented that soot (particulate) leads to heart disease and harms women more than men. (In Part Two, we consider specific health issues in the "Essential Facts and Resources for Latinas" discussions.)

Unfortunately, when you hear a report that the air quality is good, it actually means very little. It just reflects the level of six substances that are monitored by the U.S. Environmental Protection Agency (EPA). The national standards cover only carbon monoxide, lead, nitrogen dioxide, ground-level ozone, sulfur dioxide, and particulate matter. There are two kinds of particulate matter, which are measured as "very small" (PM_{10} or less then 10 micrometers in diameter) or "fine" ($PM_{2.5}$ or less then 2.5 micrometers in diameter). If you took seven particles that were the size of PM_{10} or twenty-eight that were $PM_{2.5}$, they would be just about as wide as a strand of hair. The fine particulates are now known to be more likely to harm our health.

The EPA also produces a report known as the Toxic Release Inventory. The TRI contains data on the release of 650 chemicals, but the report is released only every two years. While the TRI is not timely enough for you to do very much at the individual or community level, what it does give you is an indication of the sources of air toxics in your community. The EPA states, "The majority of air toxics come from manmade sources, such as factory smokestack emissions and motor vehicle exhaust." There are thousands of other chemicals for which there is no monitoring. Also, of increasing concern are those chemicals that, once released, tend to accumulate. The EPA refers to them as persistent bioaccumulative toxics (PBTs) because in addition to being toxic, "they remain in the environment for long periods of time, are not readily destroyed, and build up or accumulate in body tissue." Unfortunately, the EPA's way of operating makes it difficult for most of us to have clean air because a substance is not considered dangerous until it is proven to be hazardous to human health. Proving through research that something is dangerous to people can be made to drag on and on. In the meantime, the pollutant is out there for us to breathe.

WHEN THE GOAL AND THE REALITY CLASH:
The EPA's stated goal for clean air is to "protect and improve the air so it is healthy to breathe and risks to human health and the environment are reduced." The EPA recognizes "that air pollution in the form of particulate matter, or PM, at concentrations of particulate matter currently allowed by national standards (the National Ambient Air Quality Standards, or NAAQS) is linked to thousands of excess deaths and widespread health problems."

What is the EPA doing in the interim, while research is continuing? Not very much, as the actual process for enforcement lets decisions languish in a series of plans and appeals, rather than promoting timely action and saving lives.

That's why individual involvement is important. You need to know whether local toxic releases are from your local dry cleaners or from some nearby plant or facility. A federal law called the Emergency Planning and Community Right to Know Act (EPCRA) gives you the right to know about hazardous and toxic chemicals released in your community. Unfortunately, even with this law, it is hard to find out what is going on. Still, at the very least, you need to be aware of the Air Quality Index in your community and get what information you can about where your community's sources of toxic releases are. The "More Resources" listings in Part Three are guides to some good sources of information.

CLEAN INDOOR AIR

Clean indoor air is important to us all. The major way to keep the air in our homes clean is not to allow people to smoke in or near our homes, especially if we have children. The smoke from tobacco has worse effects on children because their bodies are still developing.

But sometimes we do not know when what we are breathing is not good for our lungs and the rest of our body. Radon, an odorless, tasteless gaseous substance that is naturally occurring in some parts of the country, is the leading cause of lung cancer among nonsmokers. Radon is also the second leading cause of lung cancer for all people. It is good to get a radon test kit at your local hardware store to see if your home has radon.

Volatile organic compounds (VOCs) are in many of the products we use indoors. Paint, cleaning supplies, glues and adhesives, permanent markers, copiers, and printers are just some of the products that produce VOCs. The VOCs released by some of these products stay in the air even after we have finished using them, and the EPA has documented that there are more VOCs indoors than outdoors. Research has already proven that VOCs have short- and long-term negative effects on our health. Other sources of indoor air pollution include products that you burn (oil, gas, kerosene, coal, and wood), asbestos-containing insulation, wet or damp carpet, cabinetry or furniture made of certain pressed-wood products, and household cleaning products. If you have gas appliances that are not properly adjusted, they can release carbon monoxide, which can kill you.

In houses that do not have good ventilation, some of these hazardous substances can collect to levels that are dangerous. Mold and mildew may grow in homes where there is warmth and the humidity is above 50 percent.

That smell from newly dry-cleaned clothes is perchloroethylene, which causes cancer in animals. According to the EPA,

"If dry-cleaned goods have a strong chemical odor when you pick them up, do not accept them until they have been properly dried. If goods with a chemical odor are returned to you on subsequent visits, try a different dry cleaner." Here are some more steps you can take to make sure the air in your house is clean:

- *Check the outdoor air quality before you open windows.*
- *Do not let people smoke in or near your house.*
- *Read labels and follow instructions for all products.*
- *Do not mix cleaning products, as they sometimes can form dangerous fumes. For example, do not mix chlorine-based products with other products.*
- *Get a carbon monoxide alarm if you have gas appliances.*
- *Use nonacetone products for your nails.*

CLEAN WATER

Many city dwellers think their tap water is safe to drink because public water supplies are treated. These waters are typically treated with chemicals, such as chlorine, to reduce the risks of infectious disease from waterborne pathogens.

The good news is that cleaning the water with chemicals and disinfectants is highly effective in reducing the incidence of cholera and typhoid. The not-so-good news is that sometimes these cleaning agents result in the creation of new problem substances known as disinfection by-products (DBPs). The EPA is collecting information on the effect of DBPs on humans. DBPs are known to have negative health effects in animals, and there is concern that DBPs will be associated with cancer and reproductive problems in people.

In the meantime, most of us are drinking water out of the tap. It may be a better health move to drink water that is filtered, as demonstrated by what happened in Washington, D.C.

In mid-January of 2009 the D.C. Water and Sewer Authority wrote to consumers to let them know that "during a 14 minute period on the evening of December 22, 2008 the McMillan [treatment] plant had exceeded the U.S. Environmental Protection Agency (EPA) standard for water turbidity due to a filter malfunction." The reason for the letter was that when this type of problem occurs there is a requirement by EPA under the federal Safe Drinking Water Act to notify consumers. In the same envelope there was also a January 5, 2009, news release from the U.S. Army Corps of Engineers, Baltimore District, and a December 30, 2008, letter from the Department of the Army that covered the same incident. The latter had two notable paragraphs:

> "Individuals with extremely compromised immune systems may have been at an increased risk of gastrointestinal illness. Anyone that has concerns should contact their health care provider.
>
> "Please share this information with all the other people who drink this water, especially those who may not have received this notice directly (for example people in apartments, nursing homes, schools, and businesses). You can do this by posting this notice in a public place or distributing copies by hand or mail."

Nowhere in all that correspondence had the actual time of the fourteen-minute mishap been stated, only that it had occurred on a certain "evening." But the greatest concern is that most people never even knew that the mishap had occurred.

Just as complicated as this situation has been the discussion of how much arsenic should be allowed in water. According to the EPA, "Studies have linked long-term exposure to arsenic in drinking water to cancer of the bladder, lungs, skin, kidney, nasal passages, liver, and prostate. Non-cancer effects of ingesting arsenic include cardiovascular, pulmonary, immunological, neurological, and endocrine (e.g., diabetes) effects."

According to the Natural Resources Defense Council, the total risk of cancer varies as a function of arsenic level in tap water. At 5 parts per billion (ppb) the risk is 1 in 1,000; at 10 ppb, 1 in 500; and at 20 ppb, 1 in 250. It is amazing that such tiny amounts of arsenic can have such major effects. The EPA states that 10 ppb, the current standard, is like adding "a few drops of ink in an Olympic-size swimming pool." Although an Olympic-size pool is huge—164 feet (50 meters) long, 82 feet (25 meters) wide, 6.74 feet (2 meters) deep, with a capacity for 660,430 gallons (2,500,000 liters) of water—the equivalent of those "few drops of ink" clearly can have devastating health effects. Tiny amounts of toxins can have huge health consequences.

People who use well water also need to get their water tested, since those sources also have dangerous levels of substances all too often. Whatever your water source, remember that just because water looks clean, it still may not be safe to drink. That is why you need to learn as much as you can about your own water supply.

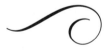

WORKING TOWARD MENTAL WELLNESS

SOMETIMES LATINAS EXPERIENCE SADNESS THAT SEEMS overwhelming and incapacitating, nervousness and anxiousness so pronounced that it is hard to get anything done, or a sense that others are out to get them. At one time Latinas were reluctant to talk about such feelings. Recent studies have shown, though, that while there is still some stigma, Latinas have become more willing to talk about their experiences and seek professional help.

In the case of depression this change is especially important, as depression has such a major impact among Latinas. The recognition that this is a treatable disease is very important. We also know that while the birth of a child is often welcomed, for some Latinas the shift in hormones and all the changes in family life can result in postpartum depression. Latinas do not have to suffer in silence. Through a combination of medication and therapy, much can be done to alleviate depression.

What is new in our understanding of mental health is the expansion of research on what makes for well-being and happiness. At the forefront of this movement is Dr. Martin Seligman, of the University of Pennsylvania. He is known as the founder of positive psychology, which focuses on "the positive emotions and character traits and the institutions that foster them."

> The practice of psychology should include an understanding
> of suffering and happiness, as well as their interaction,
> and validated interventions that both relieve suffering
> and increase happiness—two separable endeavors.
>
> —Martin E. P. Seligman, Tracy A. Steen, Nansook Park, and
> Christopher Peterson. "Positive Psychology Progress: Empirical
> Validation of Interventions" American Psychologist,
> July-August 2005 Vol. 60, No. 5, Pgs 410-421

In this new model, mental health is not just the absence of mental illness but also the presence of positive emotions and traits. The model declares that for mental health we also need to have a sense of well-being.

Some of Dr. Seligman's research findings have proven contrary to what most people might expect, especially in the area of happiness. It seems that once you have your basic needs met, more money does not bring you happiness. The same is also true for education and IQ—that is, more education does not make you happier, nor does being smarter. But happiness is an important goal for us to work toward. People who are happy have better health and are more successful.

In 2004 Dr. Christopher Peterson and Dr. Seligman took a major step in creating a classification system for the character strengths and virtues (CSVs) that are most essential to develop for our total mental wellness. In the book *Character Strengths and Virtues: A Handbook and Classification*, they identified six major virtues that we need to have in order to enjoy well-being and happiness. These virtues are classified as the "High Six": wisdom, courage, humanity, justice, temperance, and transcendence.

As Latinas, we can think about how these virtues may play out in our lives:

VIRTUES AND CHARACTER STRENGTHS

Wisdom and knowledge: creativity, curiosity (interest, novelty-seeking, openness to experience), open-mindedness (judgment, critical thinking), love of learning, and perspective (wisdom)

Courage: bravery, persistence (perseverance, industriousness), integrity (authenticity, honesty), vitality (zest, enthusiasm, vigor, and energy)

Humanity: love, kindness (generosity, nurturance, care, compassion, altruistic love, "niceness"), and social intelligence (emotional intelligence, personal intelligence)

Justice: citizenship (social responsibility, loyalty, team work), fairness, and leadership

Temperance: forgiveness and mercy, humility and modesty, prudence, and self-regulation (self-control)

Transcendence: appreciation of beauty and excellence (awe, wonder, elevation), gratitude, hope (optimism, future-mindedness, future orientation), humor (playfulness), and spirituality (religiousness, faith, purpose)

—CHRISTOPHER PETERSON AND MARTIN E. P. SELIGMAN,
CHARACTER STRENGTHS AND VIRTUES:
A HANDBOOK AND CLASSIFICATION
(OXFORD: OXFORD UNIVERSITY PRESS, 2004).

1. **Wisdom and knowledge** are not about IQ or being at the top of your class but rather your approach to learning and your ability to apply what you learn. For Latinas, we pass wisdom and knowledge from one generation to another. It is in the *dichos* (sayings) and *cuentos* (stories) we share that our struggles and

triumphs are given to the next generation as lessons. Our willingness to share and learn is a strength we can build on.

2. **Courage** is less about being the heroine and more about showing through your actions the values that drive what you do. Courage is about sticking to something until it is done, being honest about what you do, and being enthusiastic about whatever you do. Recognizing who we are as Latinas is part of our authenticity, and courage defines our *ganas* (determination and will).

3. **Humanity** is about your ability to love others, be kind, and understand what others are feeling. It is how we take care of each other. No matter how many generations we are in the United States, our sense of belonging to a common Hispanic community should be the basis of our love and appreciation for humanity. The diversity of our community and the adversity so many have to overcome should foster the development of this strength.

4. **Justice** is the underpinning of living in a community and doing what you can to make it work. Justice addresses our ability to work fairly with others and our responsibility to society as whole. Leadership, as an aspect of justice, means that you know how to motivate others to complete the necessary tasks. The Latina sense of community reflects our understanding of justice.

5. **Temperance** means that moderation is the essence of what you do. This includes the ability to move forward and not hold grudges. While you forgive others, you also recognize their personal limits. This requires that you are willing to admit your own mistakes and make amends for them. It also means you know how to restrain from following the wrong path.

6. **Transcendence** means that you are well grounded and appreciate all that surrounds you, from the exceptional to the mundane. It does not mean standing around in awe but, instead, recognizing special qualities and the connections we have to one another. This characteristic includes a sense of playfulness and optimism that includes spirituality. You understand that there is a purpose in life as a whole and in your life.

Consider these six virtues and honestly identify which are your strengths and which are the ones you need to work on. Look at the good things in your life, and try to make a regular habit of writing down and counting your blessings. Research has shown that this practice is more important than you may have ever imagined. Equally important, look at what interrupts you and gets you off track from achieving the well-being you deserve. Remember that well-being is a dynamic state involving an ongoing process. The steps you take to develop the "High Six" will help to nurture the well-being you have in your life.

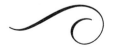

NURTURING YOUR SPIRIT THROUGH HEALTHY RELATIONSHIPS AND FAITH

O UR SPIRIT IS THE PART OF OUR LATINA ESSENCE THAT sustains us. We know that we can endure and survive. It is what gives us the strength to do what we have to do when we are too tired to even ask for help.

For some, spirit is the strength that comes from our faith, while for others it comes from a connection at a level that is beyond words. We know that spirit exists because we feel it in our quiet moments, as when we lie in bed and listen to the sounds of the night. It is that sense of spirit that unites us with one another. We may have differences, but at a basic level our struggles resonate with each other and bring us to a common ground. For some, this sense of connection is intimidating. We may want to break from our *familia*, religious traditions, and spiritual ties because these connect each one of us in ways that may be uncomfortable. But they can also be a source of strength. For Latinas, we know that healthy relationships and faith are essential to our spirit. Our sense of connectedness to our friends and family is part of who we are. We know it. We feel it. What we must do is understand how to keep these components of our spirit as a source of nurturance.

SIGNALS OF DRAINING RELATIONSHIPS

We should know when a relationship is a source of strength and when it is not. There are clear warning signs that a relationship is becoming unhealthy or draining. Here are some important cues.

Unhealthy Need.

The only needs we have are for food, water, shelter, and clothing; fulfilling those needs should not be the basis of a relationship. Healthy and meaningful relationships are born from strength and shared interests. They are based on common wants. Relationships based on need do not enhance your spirit. Instead, they bring you to an emotionally unhealthy place. When the need for a relationship becomes too great, it distorts the relationship's balance. In those instances you end up doing things you would not normally do, plus doing too much; neither is good.

Envidia.

Another sign that a relationship is not beneficial is when you either sense or feel *envidia* (envy). Somehow the word envy does not have the same connotation in English as it has in Spanish, because *envidia* has a more sinister gloss to it.

Manipulative Tears.

Whenever there are tears, you need to ask yourself what is being communicated. For Latinas, tears have always been seen as a means of expressing deep emotion. Our partner's tears have been interpreted as a sign of emotions that are deep and touch the spirit. Seeing our partner cry would make us stop whatever we were doing. But our explanations for someone else's tears may have been totally wrong.

Tears can be signs of pain, loss, joy, shame, hostility, anger, frustration, and even triumph. No single feeling can define tears. The social function of crying is to get support and sympathy from those who witness it. And it still works that way, unless we are on guard.

In her heart Yvette knew that she had been married for too long to Oscar. She knew that he would never be anything more than a man who was selfish and unloving. He had proven this to her so many times. And as difficult as it was for her to admit, Yvette could no longer be with him.

She had hoped for far too long that somehow the love and laughter that had been part of their early years together would return. Yvette was very sad when she finally decided to file for divorce, but she had accepted the truth in what her mother had always said: "Más vale sola que mal acompañada" (Better alone than with the wrong person).

When Oscar received notice of the divorce, he immediately confronted her. How could she do this? This was hurting him so deeply. How could she be so cruel? And then he began to cry. The tears moved Yvette deeply. As she looked at the face she had loved, she began to consider whether she might have been mistaken. There were still the embers of the man she knew. Perhaps with some gentleness and patience on her part he would once again be the man she had fallen in love with. The next day she saw her attorney and withdrew her request for a divorce.

It was only months later, when Oscar filed for divorce, that she realized his tears had not meant what she had thought. Oscar had cried out of sadness that he would be alone rather than sadness about losing her. He had been crying for himself.

NOURISHING FAITH PRACTICES

Along with healthy relationships, faith can play a major role in nourishing our spirit. For Latinas, faith is more important than it is for some other groups. For example, 66 percent of Hispanics attend church services at least once a month, while only 54 percent of all other Americans do. While 6 percent of Hispanics are not affiliated with any faith, 63 percent are Catholic, 16 percent are Protestant, 10 percent are other Christian affiliations, and 3 percent are of other faiths.

Whatever our choice, the faith we practice is intertwined with our spirit.

For many of us, our faith is a source of strength and renewal. Faith gives us answers when none are available otherwise. Faith sustains us during those moments when all we have is our prayers. And when it comes to our health, the good feelings that come from our prayers can be objectively monitored by tracking our brain waves.

Susana was new to our neighborhood, so I had invited her to our house for a family dinner. I couldn't help but notice that my Tia (Aunt) Consuelo had spent the night talking to Susana. I shuddered, knowing what the conversation was probably about. Tia Consuelo was very devout, and whenever possible she would talk about her faith, God, and the Virgin Mary. I didn't want Susana to feel uncomfortable, and I started apologizing for whatever Tia had said. But Susana was pleased and honored that Tia had spoken to her about those topics. Susana had been raised in a community where talking to God was an experience that many shared. It was okay with her, even though she didn't share the same beliefs.

When we care for ourselves, we nourish ourselves. While food, love, sexual intimacy, rest, and play are positive and enjoyable in our lives, they are all most beneficial in moderation. The benefits of our healthy behaviors are thrown off when we let our decision making be driven by cravings. When cravings are driving what we do, we should take that as a sign that the wrong part of our brain has been activated. Satisfying a craving or needing something to the exclusion of other aspects of our lives does not improve our health or provide nourishment.

As discussed throughout this chapter, we have many ways of caring for ourselves. We need to actively nourish ourselves through faith, relationships, sexual intimacy, healthy eating, and mental wellness. We need to stay vital by incorporating movement into our lives. And we need to be proactive to ensure that we and our communities have clean air and safe water. This means we must learn to take care of ourselves as whole people, using our unique Latina wisdom by:

1. Avoiding all smoke (first-, second-, and thirdhand smoke).
2. Going for annual wellness visits.
3. Eating good and good-for-you foods.
4. Getting fit for your heart, flexibility, and strength.
5. Sleeping soundly and sufficiently.
6. Enjoying sexual intimacy.
7. Promoting clean air and safe water.
8. Working toward mental wellness.
9. Nurturing your spirit through healthy relationships and faith.

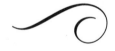

Caring for Others: Our Children, Our Partner, and Our *Familia*

CHAPTER

4

I HAVE SPENT SO MUCH TIME TALKING ABOUT THE IMPORTANCE of Latinas putting themselves first—at least *some* of the time—because doing that is the starting point for taking care of ourselves, for today and the future. But of course our *familias* are always in our minds. For many of us, taking care of others is an important part of our lives.

What you learn to do for yourself and what you do to improve your health can make a big difference in the lives of those you love. While taking good care of yourself, understanding the medical system, having regular health checkups, and nurturing yourself with good food, exercise, sleep, and sexual intimacy are good things for you, they also serve as a blueprint and guide for those around you.

A different process is involved, however, when you are responsible for someone else's health, and it is valuable to think about how the help and support you provide can make a difference in someone else's life. Here are some lessons learned from the lives of countless Latinas who are struggling to take care of their *familia* (family). Naturally, the place to start is with the health of children.

OUR CHILDREN

WHETHER OR NOT WE HAVE OUR OWN BIOLOGICAL children, we are involved in the lives of children. Sometimes when we think of the children in our lives, we feel joy, yet at other times we feel overwhelmed. It is not surprising that we can feel both emotions at the same time. For certain, raising children is hard work, no matter how much we love them or how wonderful they may be. Nevertheless, we know that whatever struggles we go through to make their lives better are worth the effort because they are the future.

THE RIGHT NUMBER

Think about these important questions: How many children do you want to have? How soon in your life and in your marriage do you and your partner want to have children? How many children can you raise, in terms of providing attention and nurturing? There is no single right answer to any of these questions. For all of us, though, deciding whether or not we want to have children and then when we do, considering what the ideal spacing between children should be are important matters that define our lives.

Our goal in raising healthy children should be simple: to help children become the best human beings they can be. That is a big challenge because many of us are still trying to address our own struggles. Raising children requires that we reach beyond our own limitations, fears, and failures. When difficulties are more than we can handle or have answers for, part of raising healthy children means we have to ask for others' help.

In the best of situations we are not alone; there are other healthy adults in the community whom we can turn to and rely on to help steer our children in the best direction. In addition to adults, other children—relatives, neighborhood playmates, and children of trusted adults—also play a role in each others' development. This is the strength of being raised in a supportive community.

For many of us, this sense of extended family is how we were raised. *Tías* (aunts), *tíos* (uncles), *comadres* (friends), *madrinas* (godmothers), *padrinos* (godfathers), *primos* (cousins), and many others formed the community in which we grew up. Some were related to us by blood or marriage, and others were connected to us by shared life experiences. The American concept of a nuclear family (father, mother, and two children) never reflected the way Hispanic communities are organized.

For those of us who are children of immigrants or are second- and third- generation Americans, we struggle to find the balance between keeping the closeness of family for our children while also creating more independence. We work to give our children the best of what is *familia* and *cultura* without the baggage that may have limited our own lives. It is very hard and demanding work because we have to put aside our own issues.

We take care of our children by starting them on the right path to having a healthy body, mind, and spirit. We teach them that good eating is important for their health, movement is central to health, clean air and water are essential and precious to life, and sexuality is part of development. In many ways these basics are the same for all of us, but when it comes to our children, we need to tailor what we teach children to their age and stage of development.

While we know that we have to start teaching children about good habits as early as possible, we know all too well that they learn most from watching others' behaviors—especially our own. This means that if we want children to brush their teeth every night before they go to sleep, we have to show them that we do it ourselves. Similarly, if we want our children not to lie to us, then we cannot lie to them. Children also have to witness that we do not lie to others.

TEN THEMES FOR NURTURING HEALTHY CHILDREN

To make our task a bit more manageable, there are ten basic themes and some tips that should help us in our work to have healthy children.

Appreciate nutritious food, safe water, and clean air.

We need to encourage children to develop taste buds that appreciate that eating food is about nutrition and energy. That is why it is good to avoid giving children food with added salt (sodium) or too much sugar. You need to redefine "treats" as something that helps children grow strong. Giving children whole fruits and vegetables helps them to appreciate these foods as the treats they should be. Being thoughtful about what you cook, eat, and serve will help children make good choices. As children get older, you can teach them how to read the labels on foods to know what they are eating.

Teaching children about the importance of safe water and clean air helps them respect our environment.

Be as physically active as possible.

According to the October 2008 report *Go Out and Play,* released in October 2008 by the Women's Sports Foundation, Latinas were the group least likely to encourage their daughters to be involved in sports. Additionally, young Latinas were the group least likely to exercise. As parents, we need to encourage, support, and model for our children the importance of physical activity. If we make this a lifelong habit for ourselves and for our children, we will be doing much to help children have a healthier life.

Visit the health care provider.

Children need to learn that going to a health care provider for wellness visits, as well as when they are ill, is something they will do for the rest of their lives. When you take children to see their health care provider, you teach them that such visits are important. You need to explain the purpose of each visit so that children begin to learn when it is good to go to a health care provider.

As children get older, you can encourage them to discuss their own health, write down any questions they may have, read the labels and instructions for their medicines (both prescription ones and over-the-counter products), and understand how their body works. By the time they are adolescents, you should encourage them to maintain a health journal and to be alone with their health care provider for part of the visit. Through these actions children learn that taking care of themselves means going for health visits, talking to the health care provider about how they feel, understanding what the health care provider says, and knowing that it is okay to ask questions.

I know that who I am today is because I had unconditional love. No matter what, I knew that they loved me. And I had that unconditional love from two people—Aunt Clara and Lucy.—Claire

Maintain a loving and safe home.

Children need to know that they are loved. We also have to balance being caring with being firm, protecting with encouraging independence, and teaching with creating opportunities for self-discovery. For example, as parents, we have to be engaged in the lives of our children and paradoxically give them space to foster their independence. At each age this means that we need to take a different approach.

When children are very young, we protect them and create a safe space for them. As they grow older, we allow and encourage them to explore on their own. Sometimes we have to allow them to fall so that they will learn how to pick themselves up. And we do all this with the gentleness that our role as parents requires. As our children get older and are able to handle more responsibility, then we can gently hand over the reins of life to them. But that transfer is a process; it does not happen at the same predetermined age for every child.

Children also need to be in a home where there is healthy resolution of conflict. This means that children need to see that when people disagree, they resolve their issues without yelling or becoming either verbally or physically abusive. There is no instance where violence in the home is acceptable. If there is violence of any kind, you must seek professional help for you and your family. Children raised in families where there is discord develop a wide array of psychological problems; and for children exposed to violence or abuse, the negative impact is magnified.

Build self-esteem.

The most important way we, as Latinas, demonstrate that we care about and love our children is by helping them develop healthy self-esteem. Children learn to value themselves when we show them that we value ourselves, them, and others. We need to show children that character strengths and virtues define not only who we, as their parents, are but also who they will become.

Too often I have heard a Latina say, "They are too little to know what's happening," even as she behaved in a way that was not in the children's best interest. In fact, quite the opposite is true. All the data show that even babies can respond to negative emotions around them. Children feel and are aware of much more than what they can express. Sometimes the way they behave reflects what they feel but cannot express.

> *Alicia came home from school so joyful because she had been chosen to play the flute. She started to play for her mother and said, "Mom, wasn't that great?" Alicia's mom paused and looked up from her computer and said, "You are a wonderful daughter, and for someone who just picked up the flute today, you are doing well." Ann frowned and said, "I thought you loved me and would tell me it was great." Her mom looked at her, smiled, and gave her a big hug as she said, "I do love you, and that is why I will always tell you the truth."*

Through what we do and say, we show children the value of having a healthy sense of self-esteem. Being a parent requires much thought because we sometimes have to keep our own feelings in check and focus on what lesson we want our child to learn. We have to think about the consequences of our own actions. We may have to manage a delicate truce between being genuine and demonstrating a healthy response. There may be times when we are furious, but our response needs to be measured to meet the child's needs. This is often tough to do, but it is the only desirable option if the goal is for our children to have a sense of security and a positive sense of self.

I know of Latinas who mistakenly think that building self-esteem means always telling your children that what they have done is great, even when that is not the case. This approach leads children in the wrong direction. What typically happens is that over time children expect enthusiastic feedback for whatever they do, no matter how small or poorly executed; they do not value feedback from their parents because it is always the same; and they do not learn that it is acceptable for them not to be great. Your feedback is best when it applauds your children's effort and their willingness to try new things, even if they do not succeed.

Self-esteem also means that we help our children have healthy boundaries in the relationships they have with us and with others. We have to be clear about the different roles each person has in their lives. While it is good to be close to our children, we also have to make it clear that we cannot be their friends because we are their parents. Unlike someone who is a friend, we parents have the job of loving them unconditionally, teaching them, saying yes and no, and being the decision maker on key choices. These are not the types of things a friend does.

By our own actions, we teach children that love is not shown by being either controlling or intrusive. That is why we give them privacy, with the understanding that privacy is a privilege to be maintained through trust and demonstrated good judgment. Sometimes it is hard to know whether children are engaged with the healthiest group of peers. The trends toward using increased text messaging, spending time on social networking sites, and meeting somewhere to go out in groups make it difficult for parents to know all of the people who influence their children. The good news is that, according to research, broad claims of harassment in social networking sites do not seem valid. When there are activities in other homes, you should feel comfortable calling the adults who will be present to understand the level of supervision they will provide and discuss what rules they will enforce.

Self-esteem also means that we need to encourage independent thinking and show that we value it. When we talk to our children and listen to what they have to say, we encourage them to talk to us. Again, the balance is to teach them what we think and correct them when they are wrong, but in a way that is informative and not devaluing or demeaning. We need to create these opportunities in all kinds of situations. This means we need to encourage children to play with others, to read by themselves, and to engage in tasks that build their exposure to the world.

Appreciate differences.
The only ideal is to be as healthy as one can be. It seems that Hispanic girls and boys are more likely to have issues with respect to body image than do other children. Healthy body awareness and acceptance are important to develop in all children.

> *The ladies at the store assumed that I did not speak Spanish. One of them looked at me and whispered to the other in Spanish, "She is so white she probably bathes in milk." I could feel my cheeks turn red in embarrassment and anger. I ran to my mother and told her what the woman had said. My mother looked at me and advised, "You should have smiled and in Spanish said, "Oh no, not milk—just soap and water like you." My mom knew the words to say to make a point at so many levels and make me feel good about myself.—Isabel*

This means that through your words and actions, you demonstrate that you value all cultures, religions, and people. The best way to do this is by never using derogatory language or telling insulting jokes about our own or other cultures. We should be proud of our Spanish language and heritage.

Exposure to degrading comments, whether in personal interactions or from other sources, is not good for anyone. For example, teens who listen to music with lyrics that are degrading and sexual are more likely to engage in early sexual behavior than teens who listen to music that have lyrics that are only sexual.

Place limits on television time and programs.
Excessive television watching should be discouraged, and we should be especially concerned with boys watching too much television, since that pattern is highly associated with depression in the future. For girls, recent studies have shown that there is a link between watching sexual content and getting pregnant before age twenty.

Liz knew that sitting and watching a movie was not something she preferred to do with her mom. They would cook, clean, shop, and do chores together because that way they could talk. It made Liz feel so special to know that her mom wanted to listen to what she had to say.

Forty years of research have confirmed that watching violent programs has a negative effect on children. These images, even when they are in the category of cartoonish or fantasy violence, increase the number of violent thoughts, behaviors, and feelings in children. Additionally, they decrease the likelihood that the children who watch such images will be helpful. What seems valuable is for parents to watch programs with their children and discuss what they are viewing.

Share accurate information about sex, sexuality, and sexual intimacy.

Talking about sex, sexuality, and sexual intimacy is not a one-time discussion. Hispanic parents need to know that these topics should be part of an ongoing conversation. We are seeing that the idea of being sexy, especially for girls as young as nine, is a growing problem. Much of it has to do with the explosion in advertising that has targeted children. In the early 1980s companies spent about $100 million to advertise to kids; by 2008 the number was $17 billion.

While much of the push to shorten childhood can be laid at the feet of advertisers, parents also have to be held accountable. We, as parents, have an important role in saying no. For instance, we have to say no to our children when they want to get clothes, screensavers, and other things that have hostile, negative, offensive, or demeaning language as well as language that is sexual.

Too many parents want to be a friend to their children. Others want so desperately to be liked by their children that they acquiesce to their children's every demand. Neither of these approaches is good. When you talk to Latinas in their late teens or early twenties, they often say that what they wanted when they were teens was to have parents who set limits.

> Boys and girls differ in how they feel about oral sex. "Boys were more likely than girls to report feeling good about themselves, experiencing popularity... whereas girls were more likely than boys to report feeling bad about themselves and feeling used."
>
> —SONYA S. BRADY AND BONNIE L. HALPERN-FELSHER, ADOLESCENTS REPORTED CONSEQUENCES OF HAVING ORAL SEX VERSUS VAGINAL SEX, *PEDIATRICS*, VOL. 119 NO. 2, PAGES 229-236, FEBRUARY 2007

It seems that for Hispanic girls the decision to have their first sexual encounter is tied to their sense of personal control and parental expectations. Young Latinas who perceived that their family thought education was important were better able to delay their sexual activity. Also, the greater the age difference between a young Latina and an older partner, the more likely she was to engage in sex at an earlier age. As parents, we need to be aware of such information and then communicate with our children.

The importance of these conversations cannot be overstated. We have to remind children that human bodies are wired to enjoy physical intimacy. What makes it difficult is that bodies develop sooner than the capacity to handle the impact of sexual intimacy—emotionally, financially, and in other ways. All the research has shown that the capacity for mature judgment does not fully develop in boys until they are in their late twenties.

So when is the right time to start talking about sex and intimacy? Probably sooner than you think. It is much harder to have these conversations if you wait until children are teenagers. You need to tailor them to the child's age and begin them before your child and her or his peers enter puberty. The facts should come from you, and you will find good articles, websites, and books at the library or bookstores to help you with these discussions.

**Discuss the facts about the abuse of
legal and illegal substances.**
Rather than focusing on messages of fear and the horrors of drugs, it is better to remind children that people who abuse drugs did not intend to end up in jail or on the street. You need to emphasize that a destructive process happens—namely, drugs take over each drug abuser's brain and entire life.

Developing faith.
Faith can give children a positive view of the future and an understanding of purposes greater than their immediate needs. It can also serve as an anchor when there is a loss in the family. Providing children with the spiritual guidance that is available through religion helps them in developing their values and getting them through the morass of conflicting social messages.

Children are healthy when we do the hard work of applying these ten themes. We want the best for our children and that means we need to be thoughtful in what we say and do.

OUR PARTNER

As LATINAS, WE TAKE CARE OF OUR PARTNER ON AN ongoing basis. In doing so, there are some specifics items that need to be part of our routine.

HEALTHY EATING

Make sure that the food in the house is healthy and tasty. The grocery list should include an assortment of vegetables, fruits, beans, whole wheat pasta, brown rice, chicken, and lean cuts of meats. If you are willing to snack on celery sticks and carrots, then have those easily accessible. If you are looking for something crunchier, have nuts, whole fruits (instead of juice), and popcorn (unbuttered). Dark chocolate in small portions (about one ounce) is also good for your heart, and it will lift your mood.

WELLNESS

Make sure that all adult vaccines are up-to-date and that you both go for annual wellness visits. Depending on your age and health history, additional annual tests and screenings may be needed. If either or both of you smoke, you need to work together to stop. Similarly, if either of you is having symptoms of depression or anxiety, it is important to see a mental health professional. Dental appointments and eye exams are also part of staying healthy. Wellness is about seeing a health care provider to avoid more serious health issues. Using the "About My Health" tools in Part Three will make those visits more fruitful. As Latinas, we have the responsibility and authority to set up the needed appointments for our partners.

MOVEMENT

Walking is a good couple activity for all ages. Finding a safe and well-lit place where you can walk is good even if you have to drive to get there. You also have the added benefit of conversation. Being active in some team activity may be another option. If one of you enjoys being on a team, the other one can be an observer or be part of the support group for the team. The goal is to get more movement in your life on a consistent basis.

SEXUAL INTIMACY

Each couple has to come to terms with what they consider to be the essential aspects of sexual intimacy and the frequency of sexual encounters. These desires go through major shifts, depending on what is going on in a couple's life. Some of these events include the birth of a child, the onset of menopause, changes in health, career shifts, financial stress, and most anything else. The reason is simple. When you are intimate with your partner, you share yourself. A person's ability to share and be intimate is a function of what is going on in her or his life.

There is great variability among Latinas regarding their desire for sexual intimacy as they go through changes in their lives. For instance, some Latinas experience menopause as a time of heightened arousal, while others seem to completely lose their desire for sexual intimacy. What is most important is that couples talk to each other when the level of sexual intimacy is not at a mutually satisfying level. If the situation becomes increasingly difficult, it is good to seek help from a health care provider.

For Latinas, taking care of the people in our lives is something we do, but we cannot care for our partner to the point of

Ana was vibrant, funny, and politically astute, and her husband was quiet, humorless, and data driven. Somehow, to the amazement of those who knew them, their life together spanned two children and two decades. And then one day when we were going to lunch, we had to go back to her house because she had forgotten her sweater. As she went upstairs, she mumbled something about "my own room" and something about how it was easier to have her own room because, that way, she could always find whatever she was looking for. I was silent and just said, "Oh of course..." as I let the full meaning of her words come to life in my mind. "My own room" meant that her husband had a different bedroom. It made me very quiet.

I asked Ana if she was happy in her marriage. Ana smiled as she stated that she had two wonderful children and that she and her husband were friends, although they had separate bedrooms. And she said she knew that after decades of marriage, friendship would be what would sustain them in their senior years. I pushed her even more and asked whether she would stay with John if she had a million dollars. Without skipping a beat, she volunteered that she would split the money with him because he had been a good father and then go off on her own. She added coyly that somewhere out there she might find the love of her life.

Seven years later John came home and announced that he preferred to be alone; he had always been a recluse, but now life had changed and he preferred that. They had been friends, he acknowledged, but he really did not want to spend the last years of his life married to anyone. Ana was surprised and hurt. Although today Ana lives by herself she still hopes she will find the love of her life.

neglecting ourselves. If we do not enjoy being with our partner, then perhaps it is time to rethink the relationship. Sometimes, after spending more time together, you find that your own and your partner's likes and dislikes have shifted.

We had waited for eight years to have a child. We talked about what it would mean to our relationship. Roberto was so enthusiastic about having a baby. He knew he was not going to be like his father. Having been raised by my mother and grandmother, I was thrilled at the thought that one day I would have a wonderful child who had a loving and attentive father.

And look at me now. Our beautiful daughter is six months old, and I feel totally overwhelmed. Is it always the woman who has to take care of everything? I work, I take care of the house, I take care of the baby, I make all the arrangements for child care, and where is Roberto? He is working late and not getting home till 10:00 p.m. He thinks he is better than his father because he changes a diaper every now and then. That is not enough. It is too much for me. I can't believe this is where we are. I would rather be alone and raise my baby by myself.—Ida

When the changes are in the same direction, then you end up in a long and happy relationship. When the changes are in different directions, then you have to reassess the relationship and determine how you are going to reconcile the differences or whether it is time to move on. In some cases you may need to seek professional help so that you can establish your own healthy boundaries.

At the most basic level you have to know whether you are in a good place with your partner. According to Dr. Dan O'Leary, SUNY Stony Brook, a renowned marriage therapist, you need to ask yourself two questions: Do you love each other? Do you enjoy a good sex life? The answers to those two questions are good indicators of whether a couple will benefit from marriage therapy. If you and your partner answer yes to both questions, then the likelihood of resolving issues is the highest; with each time you answer no, the likelihood is

How did I know that Edgar and I were perfect for each other? I have no idea. All I know is that with him I felt totally loved and completely safe. We gave each other comfort and emotional sustenance. We were together all the time without suffocating each other; we supported each other's independence. It had nothing to do with how much money we had or more accurately, how much we didn't have. I knew that as long as we were together that we would be okay. And with that came a level of sexual intimacy that I have only experienced with him.—Carolina

diminished. How would you answer those questions? How do you think your partner would answer those questions? Caring for your partner requires that you be on the same page with respect to basic questions of love and sex.

Caring needs to be given by both to each other. This is especially important during those times when the relationship is suffering from outside stress. Give and take does not mean that one is always giving and the other is always taking. Imbalances, while tolerable for a short time, become grating when they continue—even if you were once willing to accept them. When there is a predominant feeling of boredom, anger, or lack of joy, it is important to seek professional help. When you do not want to take care of a partner or doing so feels like a burden, it is time to reevaluate the relationship. Reluctance to take care of a partner may be a sign that there are other issues needing to be addressed and resolved.

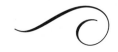

OUR *FAMILIA*

T HE OTHER ADULTS IN OUR LIVES RANGE FROM BIOLOGICAL relatives, including our parents, to those persons whom I call my life sisters and life brothers. What is a life sister? While a biological sister is one who shares the same parents, a life sister is one with whom you have shared your life experiences. This person is much more than a friend; she is someone you would trust to make end-of-life decisions for you. One way or another, life sisters and life brothers are all *familia*.

There is no other way to describe the closeness that we, as Latinas, share with those we love and the often-unspoken commitment we make to take care of them. When we take care of others in a healthy way, we are also taking care of ourselves. The challenge for us is to find the healthy balance in how we care for others so that we are neither martyrs nor saints.

Taking care of the health of our *familia* requires much of what we have already covered: eating healthily, increasing movement, encouraging regular visits to the health care provider, getting our vaccines, and so on. During different life events it also may require time that only we can give. There may be many things to do and other people to help, but in the end, we are the ones who have to put in the time. The balance and the struggle are between our need to take care of others and the need to take care of ourselves.

Throughout this book the focus has been on you because taking care of others requires taking care of yourself first. Sometimes when there is a special situation, you may have to do it all and simply focus on others. At those times you can

It was a busy time at the office, but as soon as I heard my mother had taken a turn for the worse, I flew across the continent to be with her. Taking care of my mother during those last weeks was an experience that will be with me for the rest of my life. She had been such an inspiration to me all of her life. Here she was in her nineties and she still had that gentle way about her. Yes, she was in a coma, but sometimes I knew she could hear me and respond. Once when I told her that I was going to put cream on her face, she smiled and raised her face and gave me her cheek so that she could feel the moisture. It reaffirmed that she was still with me; I still had not lost her. I was with her till the very end, and I treasure every moment that I was able to be with her, especially that last smile.—Esther

rely on your emotional, physical, and spiritual reserves to help you through. But even then, those reserves must be replenished; you cannot neglect yourself. You need to see your health care provider, get enough sleep, eat adequate food, stay fit, and get the nurturance that comes from emotional and sexual intimacy.

To take care of your children, partner, and *familia*, first and foremost you must take care of yourself.

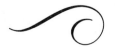

TAKING CARE OF
OUR HEALTH NEEDS

Part Two

CHOOSING WHAT TO INCLUDE IN THIS PART OF THE BOOK was challenging. There is so much health information, and I knew I could not include everything and did not want to try being exhaustive. The decision about what topics to include was driven by two considerations. First, I wanted to discuss all the diseases and health issues for which Latinas have high rates (e.g., depression, diabetes, arthritis). Second, I wanted to cover specific areas that Latinas have asked me to discuss (e.g., menstruation, sex, sexuality, and sexual intimacy). I decided also to include a "Glossary of Frequently Used Words," which appears at the end of Part Two.

Essential Facts and Resources for Latinas

Each topic is presented with the key facts, the causes, and the steps for prevention, as well as web resources to get more information. I narrowed the web resources to those that provide scientifically sound information and that are not trying to sell a product.

Of course, if you also want to talk to someone, I encourage you to call the *Su Familia* National Hispanic Family Health Helpline at 1-866-783-2645 or 1-866-Su-Familia on Monday through Friday, 9:00 a.m. to 6:00 p.m., Eastern Standard Time. The health promotion advisors who answer the phones are committed to helping you and your family stay as healthy as possible.

Alcohol Use and Alcoholism

"She's not drinking; she's just happy."

LATINAS AND ALCOHOL

- *Younger Latinas are more likely to drink a lot at one time (heavily).*
- *Latinas who are more "mainstream" are more likely to drink a lot at one time (heavily).*
- *Latinas are more likely to die of chronic liver disease and cirrhosis than other women.*
- *Latinas are less likely to know that beer is alcohol.*

Q *Que pasa?*
For most Latinas, drinking a glass of wine occasionally is not a problem. What we do know is that drinking more than seven drinks in a week or more than three drinks on any one day, is more likely to be a sign that drinking is becoming a problem. When Latinas drink too much, the drinking can lead to alcohol abuse and eventually alcoholism, the disease in which your body becomes dependent on alcohol. No one who drinks intends to become an alcoholic. Alcoholism is a disease in which the need to drink takes over someone's thinking, and as a result, the person can no longer make reasonable judgments. All the person wants to do is get another drink.

Researchers used to believe that when someone drank, the "pleasure center" of the brain was activated. We now know that the "craving" part of the brain is what gets activated. Over time a person's body tells her or his brain that it "craves" more alcohol, even though there is more damage to the body with each drink.

How does someone know how much alcohol is too much? Like most things, this varies from person to person. "Too much" depends on whether you are a man or a woman, how old you are, how much you weigh, and many other factors. For some Latinas, it is okay to have no more than seven drinks over a one-week period; for others, that may be too much. For example, some Latinas do not have the enzyme to properly process alcohol in their stomach. Those Latinas may get an "allergic" reaction to one glass of wine, such as their face turning red.

The question of "how much" is surrounded by a lot of myths that can take you in the wrong direction. While some Latinas are proud that they can "hold their liquor" and not be visibly drunk, the ability to do so is actually a sign that there may be problems ahead. The science tells us that the ability to drink and "handle it" actually increases your risk for becoming dependent on alcohol. Although you may not feel the damage that is being done to your brain and body, the damage is occurring. It is important to know that we women cannot "drink like a man" or have as much to drink as men because our bodies do not use alcohol in the same way as men's bodies do. As a result, not only are the negative impacts of drinking greater on women than on men, but they also occur sooner.

When you drink too much, there are harmful physical effects on your liver, heart, and brain. Latinas who are heavy drinkers (more than seven drinks a week) are more likely to have cancer, heart disease, and liver disease; to die from cir-

HEALTH POINT

If you are pregnant or intend to get pregnant, do not drink any alcohol.

rhosis; and to experience a decrease in brain size and functioning. But alcohol destroys more than the body.

At the emotional and spiritual levels, drinking to excess compromises our relationships with those closest to us and sacrifices our work. Additionally, drinking too much results in poor judgments (e.g., This is not a risky situation) and poor decisions (e.g., I can drive). Alcohol changes what you do and how you think.

The younger you are when you drink, the more physical damage the alcohol causes to your body and brain. Your relationships suffer, too. If you are a young Latina who drinks too much, you are more likely to end up in risky or dangerous situations. What does that mean? You may, for example, drive and end up in an accident in which someone gets hurt. Or you may wake up and realize that you have hooked up with someone you do not particularly even like or that you had sex and did not use a condom. We also know that women who are heavy drinkers—whatever their age—are more likely to be victims of violence and sexual assault, as others take advantage of the situation.

CAUSES AND PREVENTION

While there is no single cause for abusing alcohol or becoming dependent on alcohol, there are some steps you can take to avoid drinking dangerously:

1. Avoid people who drink in excess; they encourage what you are trying to avoid.
2. Do not drink when you are alone.
3. Do not take part in binge or excessive drinking for "special" events or celebrations.
4. Limit yourself to no more than seven drinks a week and no more than three drinks on any single day.

HEALTH POINT

One drink =

5 ounces of table wine (about 12% alcohol);

OR

12 ounces of regular beer (about 5% alcohol);

OR

8-9 ounces of malt liquor (about 7% alcohol);

OR

a shot (1.5 ounces) of rum, vodka, whiskey, or other hard liquor (80 proof, which is about 40% alcohol).

Read the label to know the amount of alcohol, since it can vary by type of drink.

5. Offer to be the "safe driver," thus avoiding alcohol altogether on certain days and occasions.
6. Remember that you want to keep your body healthy.
7. Remember that having family members who abuse alcohol does not mean that it is inevitable that you will also abuse alcohol.

Q Do I have a problem?

Most of the time, the person who has a drinking problem is the last one to admit that she or he drinks too much or that drinking is causing personal problems.

MYTH: You can look at people and know if they have been drinking.
FACT: It's not that easy.

MYTH: If I add juice to hard liquor, it reduces the alcohol.
FACT: The amount of alcohol remains the same.

MYTH: I drink a lot because wanting to is in my genes.
FACT: Genes may put you at risk, but it is what you do that makes the risk a reality.

Think about yourself and honestly answer the following questions:

1. Are you happy about getting wasted?
2. Have you been missing work on Monday because you partied during the weekend?
3. Do you need a drink "to smooth out the edges" or to "feel comfortable"?

4. Do you look forward to getting together with friends because everyone drinks?
5. Do you plan your day around activities that include drinking?
6. Do you sometimes hide the fact that you are drinking?
7. Do you spend time with people who drink a lot at one time?
8. Have you ever felt bad about your drinking?
9. Do you drink when you are alone?
10. Do you find that a drink in the morning helps you start the day?

If you answered yes to at least one of these questions, you may be going down a path that leads to alcoholism.

Q Can I get better?

Yes. Regardless of how desperate you may feel, by admitting that you have a drinking problem, you are taking a major step toward getting better. Many Latinas try to hide what they fear. For others, feelings of *vergüenza* (shame) may be overwhelming. Use your *vergüenza* to move you in the right direction, and seek professional help. Talk to your health care provider about treatment, which will depend on how much you are drinking and how often you drink. With treatment you will be able to enjoy life and have healthier relationships. You will have to work at the recovery process and it may be difficult at first, but the rewards will be enormous. Do not give up if treatment does not work immediately or if you have to go into treatment several times. Recovery is a process and takes commitment, time, and effort.

Q What if someone I care about has an alcohol problem?

As you may already know, a person who is abusing alcohol may seem charming and personable in the beginning.

But over time, that person's behavior changes as the dependence on alcohol increases. It is very hard when someone you know drinks to excess. If you are in this situation, seek professional help for the person and for yourself. Alcoholism is a serious disease; you cannot deal with this disease by yourself.

WHERE TO LEARN MORE

NATIONAL INSTITUTE ON ALCOHOL ABUSE AND ALCOHOLISM
   www.niaaa.nih.gov
With a range of resources, this website can be a bit technical, but it is full of helpful information.

NATIONAL LIBRARY OF MEDICINE (NLM): MEDLINEPLUS
   www.nlm.nih.gov/medlineplus/alcoholism.html
The NLM is the library resource of the National Institutes of Health, and it has an alcoholism web directory organized by topic. This site includes general information, research findings, organizations, information related to genetics, and more.

Arthritis

"Why is she complaining? We all have pain."

LATINAS AND ARTHRITIS

- *Overweight Latinas are likely to have osteoarthritis in their knees.*
- *Latinas who are active have less risk of developing osteoarthritis.*
- *Latinas are less likely to say that a health professional told them that they have some form of arthritis, rheumatoid arthritis, gout, lupus, or fibromyalgia.*
- *Latinas are more likely to suffer from arthritis than are Hispanic or non-Hispanic black men.*

Q *Que pasa?*
No one should have to live with pain. Many of us have watched as a family member said, *"Tengo artritis* (I have arthritis)," while grimacing with movements. *Aguantando* (accepting the pain) is not what either we or our family members should do. Too many of us accept the idea that the pain we have is just one more of life's hardships or a "natural" part of getting older. But pain in our bodies is not something to ignore. It is a signal we must learn to listen to. With proper diagnosis of the cause of pain, we can reduce it and do the things we want to do.

Too often the word *arthritis* is used as a catchall for the aches and pains in the parts of the body where a joint connects two bones, such as knees, wrists, fingers, shoulders, neck, back, and hips. The pain may be caused by joint inflammation or the wear and tear of a joint, or it may be an indication that your immune system is not working properly.

> **MYTH:** No pain, no gain
> **FACT:** Pain is the way your body signals that what you are doing is not good for you. When you have joint pain, you should stop what you are doing.

Wear and tear. The most common type of arthritis is osteoarthritis, which is due to wear and tear of the joint and may also come with age. How does it come about? Think about your activities and the injuries you had that went untreated because they got better on their own. An injury to your knee or some other joint may have healed quickly and felt better, but as you get older, the area that was injured is more likely to develop osteoarthritis. Additionally, as your weight increases, you are more likely to have osteoarthritis.

If you think about the words *wear and tear*, it is clear why each pound of extra weight is like four pounds of extra stress on your knees. The wear and tear on your body is not just from things such as car accidents and injuries but also from work, sports, and even the wrong type of exercise. It can even be from wearing three-inch spike heels (so just imagine what happens with four-inch ones). One thing you can do to help your joints is to be thoughtful about how you move. Movement that involves pounding of your joints should be avoided. This covers the gamut from activities that require repetition of a strenuous movement to running on cement. If your work requires any such movements, then you should regularly wear proper shoes and take rest periods.

Immune system. Sometimes the aches and pains are only part of the picture. You may also have a fever, feel tired, lose weight when you have not been trying to, have trouble breathing, and get a rash or itch. Rheumatoid arthritis, juvenile rheumatoid

HEALTH POINT

The risk, by weight, for developing osteoarthritis:

- normal weight, 35%
- overweight, 44%;
- obese, 65%.

117

arthritis, gout, lupus, and fibromyalgia are just some of the diseases that have joint pain as a symptom. In these diseases the immune system is not doing its job; instead of protecting the body, the immune system attacks it. This is why these are called autoimmune diseases. Very often these diseases also affect the heart, kidneys, skin, and other organs. Women are more likely to have autoimmune diseases. Rheumatoid arthritis is the most common of the autoimmune diseases.

CAUSES

We do not know for sure what causes all of the diseases that have swollen joints as a symptom. At this point there is very little evidence to suggest a genetic component.

HEALTH POINT

Smoking increases the risk of developing rheumatoid arthritis. Also, smokers with osteoarthritis have twice as much cartilage loss in their knees.

Q Do I have a problem?
Arthritis is not something you can diagnose yourself. Your *comadre* may be wise in so many ways, but only a health care provider can tell you what is causing the pain in your joints. If you do not have a health care provider (one-third of Latinas do not), call the *Su Familia* Helpline (1-866-SU-FAMILIA or 1-866-783-2645) to be referred to a local clinic. Once your health care provider determines the reason for your aches and pains, he or she will be able to discuss with you the treatments available to reduce pain and increase the ease with which you can move.

Q Can I get better?
At the very least, your health care provider will discuss with you what prescription and over-the-counter medicines are available and how you would need to take them. That professional can also guide you on the kinds of exercises that will help you maintain your strength and flexibility, as well as the actions you can take to maintain a healthy weight.

It is important to see your health care provider on a regular basis and to do exercises that are consistent with your diagnosis. If you have osteoarthritis, the right kinds of exercises will help to stretch and strengthen your hips, thighs, and knees. Such exercises will be important in helping you maintain a good range of motion for your legs and hips.

WHERE TO LEARN MORE

Anytime that pain is involved and you are desperate to get relief, you have to be extra careful with the websites you use, because there are companies that engage in health fraud. The following are particularly helpful and reliable resources.

NATIONAL INSTITUTE ON ARTHRITIS AND MUSCULOSKELETAL AND SKIN DISEASES
www.niams.nih.gov
The NIAMSD is part of the National Institutes of Health, and the website information includes the most up-to-date research and credible consumer guidelines.

CENTERS FOR DISEASE CONTROL AND PREVENTION (CDC)
www.cdc.gov/arthritis
The CDC's website includes extensive Arthritis Program information.

ARTHRITIS FOUNDATION
www.arthritis.org
This not-for-profit organization is an exceptional source of information and support to those who want to learn about the many diseases that are clustered under the term *arthritis*.

Asthma

*"She's just too emotional.
There is nothing wrong with her."*

LATINAS AND ASTHMA

- *Asthma is more common in women than in men.*

- *Hispanic adults have lower rates of asthma than do non-Hispanic white adults.*

- *Latinas who live in border areas have higher rates of asthma.*

- *There is very little information on how common asthma is among Hispanic adults in the United States and throughout Latin America.*

Q *Que pasa?*

Asthma is a disease of the lungs. While you can get asthma at any age, it usually starts when you are a child. Once you have asthma, you will have it for the rest of your life, although with treatment and care the symptoms can diminish.

When you have asthma, your airways (the tubes that carry air to and from your lungs) get inflamed and, as a result, get narrower, making it hard to breathe. As the airways get more inflamed, they may produce more mucus. This makes it even harder to breathe.

Besides having trouble breathing, some people may make a wheezing sound (a high-pitched whistling sound that seems to come from the chest), feel short of breath, have tightness in

> **MYTH:** More and more people are dying from asthma.
> **FACT:** While more people are getting asthma, the number of those dying is going down, since there are now better ways to manage the disease.
>
> ---
>
> **MYTH:** To prevent getting asthma, you need to make sure you take ten deep breaths of clean air every morning.
> **FACT:** There is no way to prevent getting asthma.

the chest, or cough. Not everyone has these symptoms, and sometimes these may be symptoms of some other condition. Only a health care provider can diagnose whether breathing problems are asthma.

The inflammation of the airways is how the body responds to a trigger. According to the NIAID (National Institute of Allergy and Infectious Diseases), triggers include infectious agents (such as viruses and bacteria), stress, hazardous air pollutants (including smoke from tobacco), and other common allergens (cat dander, dust mites, and pollen).

CAUSES AND PREVENTION

There is no cure for asthma, and at this time there is no way to prevent getting asthma. You can prevent asthma attacks by avoiding those substances that trigger an attack and by taking your medicines.

Q How do I control it and get better?
Once you have been diagnosed with asthma, you will be taught how to control it. You will learn to be aware of when you are getting symptoms so that they do not get worse and become asthma attacks or flare-ups.

There is much you can do to prevent having asthma attacks:

- *Be sure to develop and follow the plan that your health care provider creates with you.*
- *Take your medications as recommended by your health care provider.*
- *Track how your lungs are working by using your peak flow meter (a device your health care provider will give you) and by writing down your results.*
- *Avoid all types of hazardous air pollutants. When the air quality is poor, be sure to limit outside activities. Listen to the radio or check online to see what the air quality is in your community.*
- *Be very careful not to inhale the fumes from products used for cleaning. Some cleaning products that are considered mild in toxicity have been found to trigger respiratory symptoms in women, whether or not they have asthma.*
- *Be aware of what triggers your asthma, and avoid those substances or situations.*

HEALTH POINT

Asthma accounts for 25 percent of all emergency room visits in the United States.

Q *Can I get better?*
Most definitely. Asthma is a chronic disease that can be managed. Unfortunately, it seems that even when Hispanic children with persistent asthma have insurance, they were less likely than non-Hispanic white children to be managing their condition. We can only assume the same with adults. All the research shows that if you take your medicines, it is less likely that you will end up in the hospital or the emergency room.

Q *What if someone I know has asthma?*
People with asthma have a disease that will be with them for the rest of their lives. You can help them avoid asthma triggers.

Where to learn more

National Heart, Lung, and Blood Institute (NHLBI)
  www.nhlbi.nih.gov
The NHLBI is part of the National Institutes of Health, and it is the primary NIH organization doing research on asthma.

National Library of Medicine: MedlinePlus
  www.nlm.nih.gov/medlineplus/asthma.htm
The NLM is the library resource for the NIH, and it has some information on asthma.

Environmental Protection Agency (EPA)
  www.epa.gov/asthma/
The EPA has information on how consumers can manage their environment to reduce or eliminate triggers for asthma.

National Institute of Allergy and Infectious Diseases
  www3.niaid.nih.gov/topics/asthma
The NIAID is part of the National Institutes of Health, and it provides good consumer information on asthma.

Asthma and Allergy Foundation of America
  www.aafa.org/
The AAFA's information about asthma is for consumers.

Asthma—CDC
  www.cdc.gov/asthma/
This is the "asthma" home page for the CDC's National Asthma Control Program.

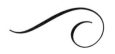

Birth Control

*"I can't believe I'm pregnant again!
How could this have happened?"*

Q *Que pasa?*
Birth control, also known as contraception, is designed to prevent or delay pregnancy. As soon as each Latina becomes sexually active, she has to make decisions about her sexual activity and birth control until she reaches the post-menopausal point in her life. Research has shown, though, that Latinas are less likely than other women to use birth control when they first become sexually active.

For those Latinas who are sexually intimate with a man, the only method for birth control that is 100 percent safe and effective is abstinence from vaginal sex, but that option is not acceptable to most Latinas. There are serious trade-offs and considerations in deciding what to do about contraception. Each woman must consider issues of safety, effectiveness, ease of use, family medical history, and other effects on her body.

Unfortunately, decades of research on the various options for birth control have not proven as helpful as should be the case. There is no method that is both 100 percent effective and risk free. Your religious and personal beliefs are a major factor in what you decide to do. It may be that at different points in your life you will choose to use a method that is more consistent with your life at that time. For example, once you have had as many children as you would like, then you might choose to undergo tubal ligation or your partner might choose to have a vasectomy. (The specific methods are described in the following discussion.)

> **MYTH:** When you are breastfeeding, you cannot get pregnant.
>
> **FACT:** You can still get pregnant.
>
> ───────────────
>
> **MYTH:** Latina teens do not talk to their parents about their sexual activity.
>
> **FACT:** Over half of the parents of Latina teens know that their daughters are going for sexual health services.

Birth control can be either temporary or permanent. Temporary methods work by preventing sperm from reaching the uterus, preventing implantation of a fertilized egg in the uterus, or preventing ovulation. Here is a summary for each of these:

STOPPING SPERM (TEMPORARY METHOD)

- *Either a cervical cap with a spermicide (a substance that destroys sperm) or a spermicide alone is about 80 percent effective, which means that one out of five times either of these will not be effective. Using either of these methods is messy, and spermicides can irritate vaginal tissue.*

- *With typical use, condoms (male and female), diaphragms, and sponges are 81 percent to 90 percent effective, which means one to two times out of ten any of these would not be effective. These methods are more effective with perfect and consistent use. Condoms provide the additional benefit of some protection from sexually transmitted diseases (STDs). The diaphragm also offers some protection from STDs but not from HIV.*

- *Copper intrauterine devices (IUDs) are 99 percent or more effective. They work by creating an environment hostile to both sperm and egg. Your health care provider must put the device in*

HEALTH POINT

Due to its high failure rate, withdrawal is not an acceptable birth control method.

125

your uterus, and she or he must also remove it. With an IUD you must monitor its placement at least once a month. With the copper IUD some women experience cramping and increased monthly bleeding during the first few months. This device works for ten to twelve years. If you are allergic to copper, you should not use the copper IUD. Another intrauterine device is the Mirena™ coil system (levongorgestrel intrauterine system, or LNG IUS), which releases progestogen (a progesterone-like substance) and is 99 percent or more effective. This device should be replaced after five years. You should not use any of these devices if you have an abnormal uterus; an artificial heart valve; a recent history of pelvic inflammatory disease or STDs; or cervical, endometrial, or ovarian cancer that needs treatment.

HEALTH POINT

In one study, females who were on birth control pills picked different types of mates than they did when they were not taking birth control pills.

CONTROLLING OVULATION (TEMPORARY METHODS)

- *Methods that involve changing the hormonal balance in your body and thereby controlling ovulation (the release of an egg) include birth control pills, birth control shots, birth control patches, and vaginal rings. All of these are 91 percent to 99 percent effective.*

   Since most women who take birth control pills continue using them for a number of years, it is important to have more research on the long-term effects of these pills, which create chemically induced periods. According to a recent report in the Journal of the American College of Cardiology, *the new versions of birth control pills do not seem to raise the risk of heart disease as much as older ones did. We do know, however, that birth control pills can increase cholesterol levels and blood pressure.*

Some women take birth control pills to avoid going through menopause. But you cannot avoid menopause. Women on birth control pills still go through menopause, but they may not know that their periods have actually stopped as they may still have periods that are chemically induced by the birth control pills.

• For the "rhythm method" (timing vaginal intercourse to avoid the days near ovulation) or other strategies based on your awareness of when you are ovulating, you have to maintain detailed records of your menstrual cycle. These methods are only about 80 percent effective.

TUBAL LIGATION AND VASECTOMY
(PERMANENT, OR IRREVERSIBLE, METHODS)

• Tubal ligation is surgery that closes the fallopian tubes (through which eggs move from the ovaries to the uterus), so that a woman cannot get pregnant. In rare occasions this can be reversed. This procedure is three times more common than vasectomy.

• Vasectomy is surgery that closes the vas deferens (sperm-carrying tubes), and it is the safest and most inexpensive option for permanent sterilization. This procedure is not reversible, except in very exceptional cases. Men who choose vasectomy do so because they recognize that this is the best way not to have any more children.

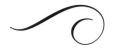

WHERE TO LEARN MORE

NATIONAL INSTITUTE OF CHILD HEALTH AND HUMAN DEVELOPMENT (NICHD)
www.nichd.nih.gov/health/topics/contraception.cfm
The NICHD is part of the NIH, and up -to-date information is available on this website.

OFFICE ON WOMEN'S HEALTH
www.4woman.gov
Birth control information from more than forty sources is available on this site.

ASSOCIATION OF REPRODUCTIVE HEALTH PROFESSIONALS (ARHP)
www.arhp.org
This membership association for physicians, nurses, public health professionals, health educators, and related professions provides a wealth of information on reproductive health.

Cancer

"Don't even say it!"

LATINAS AND CANCER

- After heart disease, cancer is the second leading cause of death (20 percent) among Hispanics.
- Latinas are less likely than non-Hispanic white women to get breast, lung, or colorectal cancer.
- Latinas are diagnosed for breast cancer at a younger age.
- Latinas are more likely than non-Hispanic white women to get skin, liver, pancreatic, or stomach cancer.
- About one in seven Latinas will get cervical cancer.
- Latinas who get cancer are less likely to survive than are non-Hispanic white women.
- Compared to non-Hispanic white women, Latinas are less likely to get diagnosed early and, consequently, more likely to be diagnosed with a more advanced stage of cancer.

Que pasa?
Sometimes our bodies have growths that are called tumors, and some of these can be harmless (benign). Examples of benign tumors are cysts and polyps, and these are located in one part of your body and stay there. Tumors that have abnormal growth and invade nearby tissue are called malignant. Although they start out in one part of the body, they may also be found in other parts of the body. *Cancer* is the term used to describe when something triggers cells in the body to multiply and grow so that they harm you.

129

Cancer is not one disease but many diseases. According to the National Cancer Institute, these are the main types of cancer:

1. Carcinoma starts in skin or in tissues that line or cover internal organs.
2. Sarcoma starts in bone, cartilage, fat, muscle, blood vessels, or other connective or supportive tissue.
3. Leukemia starts in blood-forming tissue such as the bone marrow, and it causes large numbers of abnormal blood cells to be produced and to enter the blood.
4. Lymphoma and multiple myeloma start in the cells of the immune system.
5. Central nervous system cancers start in the tissues of the brain and spinal cord.

MYTH: Only smokers get lung cancer.
FACT: Women who are nonsmokers also get lung cancer.

MYTH: If you have cancer and it spreads, you are in the more advanced stages of cancer.
FACT: There is increasing evidence that cancer cells travel to other parts of the body and go undetected until some genetic change occurs and makes them malignant.

Cancer is designated as a certain type on the basis of the primary site where it started. For example, if someone has lung cancer, it is still called lung cancer even when it has spread to other parts of the body. *Metastases* is another word used for cancer cells that have been found in other parts of the body besides the original place. Whether cancer cells have spread is information that will help your health care provider determine the best treatment options. That is why your health care provider may order a variety of tests if you have been found to have cancer. Once these tests are completed, the cancer will be described in stages, which are designated from I to IV. (Roman numerals are typically used for this purpose.) Stage I cancer has spread the least, and Stage IV cancer occurs in organs far from the original site.

CAUSES AND PREVENTION

Scientists know that many different things can make cancer cells in your body grow. Some of these triggers include exposure to toxic substances (e.g., tobacco, radon, pollutants, chemicals), viruses (e.g., the HPV virus that causes cervical cancer), and excessive exposure to sunlight. There are steps you can take to reduce the risk of turning on the cells that can turn into cancer.

1. Eliminate your exposure to hazardous substances, starting with tobacco. Firsthand smoke (when you smoke), second-hand smoke (when you are near people who are smoking), and thirdhand smoke (the smell that lingers after people have smoked) are all associated with increasing the risk for lung, breast, cervical, and prostate cancer, plus many other types of cancer. Other hazardous substances include radon, dioxin, some pesticides and disinfectants, and some cleaning products when not properly used. Be sure to read labels carefully and use the products as directed.

2. Avoid excessive exposure to radiation. The U.S. Environmental Protection Agency (EPA) is revising the criteria for how much radiation is too much for women. As of 2009, the EPA was still defining excessive exposure to radiation by using the 1975 model of a "reference man" (a supposedly average man who represents all adults)—namely, a five-foot seven-inch tall, 154-pound man "western European or North American in habitat and custom." The evidence suggests that using the same standard for women is wrong because women are 52

HEALTH POINT

Early screening increases the likelihood that you will survive.

131

percent more likely than men to get cancer if they follow the exposure guidelines based on this model.

3. If there is a vaccine to protect you from getting a type of cancer, you should consider getting it. There is now a vaccine that will protect you against cervical cancer.

4. If you are going to be in the sun, wear a hat and a shirt, and be sure to use sunscreen. The level of skin protection in your sunscreen should be at least at 30 SPF (sun protection factor), and you should put the sunscreen on as often and as thickly as recommended in the instructions or by your health care provider.

5. Talk to your health care provider about the risks and benefits of menopausal hormone therapy if you experience menopausal symptoms. Short-term use may be beneficial enough to outweigh the potential risks for you.

6. Be careful about the use of supplements. Increasingly, they are being found to contain substances that are harmful to you. Supplements are not required to meet the same standards for manufacturing, effectiveness, and safety as prescription medicines.

You can also protect yourself by going for regular screenings to detect the earliest signs that you may get cancer.

Pap test to detect cervical cancer. Getting a Pap test on a regular basis is very important for your health. With the Pap test it is possible to detect cells that are in the earliest stages of going through abnormal changes. It is at this precancerous stage that you and your health care provider will have the greatest success in stopping the cells from developing into cancer. Young women who have had sexual intercourse and all women over twenty-one should get Pap tests on a regular basis. At age sixty-five, though, you need to talk to your health care provider to discuss whether getting Pap tests less frequently would be fine.

Mammogram to detect breast cancer. While you may do your own breast exam on a regular basis, it is important to have your health care provider give you one, too. Once you are forty, you will need to have regular imaging of your breasts through mammograms or other techniques. Depending on you and your family history, your health care provider will decide what type of breast imaging is best for you, as well as how often you need to have certain imaging.

Colonoscopy to detect colorectal cancer. A colonoscopy provides a method for early detection of growths in your colon (the lower part of your large intestine) that are likely to turn into cancer. In order to take a good image, your colon (or bowel) has to be clean. Your health care provider will give you special pills or liquids to drink that will cleanse your colon. Since these work as powerful laxatives, the preparatory effects are the most unpleasant part of having a colonoscopy. When the procedure is actually done, you will be sedated. Sometimes during the procedure polyps are detected and your health care provider may remove and have them examined to determine whether they are benign or precancerous. After the colonoscopy your health care provider will explain what was found. In most cases you will be given pictures of your colon so you can see that the tissue is clean and smooth (and amazingly pink and clear).

Q Do I have a problem?
If you are diagnosed with cancer, your health care provider will probably want you to undergo further tests to determine the type of tumor you have, plus other relat-

ed tests may be needed. You may be referred to an oncologist, meaning a health care provider who specializes in treating cancer. Some medicines are more successful with some types of tumors, and other medicines are better for people who have a particular genetic pattern.

Because you may feel scared after getting a cancer diagnosis, it will be good for you to have someone go with you to take notes when you visit your health care provider, especially regarding what things you will need to do. Be sure you understand everything that is being explained to you. It is good to keep a list of each health care provider you meet with and what each tells you to do. Do not rely on your memory.

Q *Can I get better?*
Yes, you can get better. With early detection there is treatment for most cancers. Also, there are many new kinds of treatments, and increasingly treatments are being personalized to improve the success and decrease the side effects. Even if cancer is at a very advanced stage, there may be opportunities for you to be part of a clinical trial involving different treatments that are being developed.

Q *What if someone I know has cancer?*
Each person handles the diagnosis and treatment of cancer in a way that makes it easier for her or him to cope. You can offer to drive, do grocery shopping, do some regular chore, or make phone calls. Let the person who has cancer tell you what she or he needs. Some Latinas will choose to join a support group and take part in races to support persons who have also survived; others will want to go through treatment, put the whole experience behind them, and move forward to the next chapter in their lives. All you can do is support whatever the person wants to do.

WHERE TO LEARN MORE

NATIONAL CANCER INSTITUTE (NCI)
www.cancer.gov/cancertopics
The NCI, part of the National Institutes of Health, provides information on cancer treatment, prevention, screening, genetics, causes, and ways of coping with cancer.

NATIONAL LIBRARY OF MEDICINE (NLM): MEDLINEPLUS
www.nlm.nih.gov/medlineplus/cancer.html
The NLM is the library resource for the NIH, and it provides information about cancer in general, treatments, symptoms, disease management, and sources of clinical trials.

CDC: CANCER PREVENTION AND CONTROL
www.cdc.gov/cancer
The CDC works with national organizations, state health agencies, and other key groups in the prevention and control of cancer.

AMERICAN CANCER SOCIETY
www.cancer.org
As reflected on its website, the ACS is dedicated to helping everyone who faces cancer. It promotes research, patient services, early detection, treatment, and education.

LANCE ARMSTRONG FOUNDATION
www.livestrong.org
This foundation educates survivors, families, and caregivers.

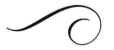

Depression

"Just get over it; it's all in your head."

LATINAS AND DEPRESSION

- *Latinas have higher rates of depression than do non-Hispanic white women.*

- *Latinas younger than eighteen have the highest rates of attempted suicide of all U.S. girls in this age group.*

Q *Que pasa?*
Depression is a disease for which there is treatment. It is not something that people can just pull themselves out of or "just get over." Getting better requires seeking treatment, just as with any other medical condition.

CAUSES AND PREVENTION

There is no single cause for depression. The National Institute for Mental Health (part of the National Institutes of Health) has stated that depression results from a combination of genetic, biochemical, environmental, and psychological factors. These factors combine in different ways for each affected individual. Although depression may be triggered by a specific event, there are many possible triggers and they vary from person to person. That is why if a group of people were exposed to the same situation, some of the people would become depressed and others would not.

At one time depression was believed to have a strong genetic component, even though there are people with depression

> **MYTH:** Depression begins once you are older than twenty-one and have increased responsibilities.
> **FACT:** Depression affects people of all ages—children, teens, adults, and seniors.
>
> ---
>
> **MYTH:** Latinas who give birth are joyful—more than other women who don't have our sense of family.
> **FACT:** Latinas also experience depression after childbirth (postpartum depression).

who do not know of any family members who have had it. Recent evidence has suggested that any existing genetic component is relatively less significant than other factors and that all of the many contributing factors must be considered.

Q *Do I have a problem?*
It is natural to feel sad because someone close to you died, you are going through a separation or divorce, or some other difficult events are going on in your life. Feeling sad some of the time is simply part of life; no one is happy all of the time. Depression is when the feelings of sadness take over your life and last for a few weeks or more instead of for a few days.

People who are depressed usually do not enjoy the activities that once gave them pleasure in the past; they also feel sad and look sad. They feel that nothing is going to get better in their lives, and their outlook becomes negative. Some people with depression also question how much they contribute to the life around them, and they feel guilty about not doing enough.

As the chains of depression hold them in an uncomfortable place, people who are depressed sometimes become particularly cranky or irritable. People who are depressed also experience changes in how much they eat and how much they sleep. Some people who are depressed eat more than usual, while others eat less. Part of the criteria for the diagnosis of depression is based on whether people are experiencing changes in their regular patterns of eating and sleeping that are not due to external causes (e.g., a change in work shift).

When reading the following checklist, you will find that some of the statements describe how you (or someone you know) may have felt at one time or another.

HEALTH POINT

Early treatment of depression is more effective than later treatment, and it reduces the likelihood that depression will occur again.

☐ *You feel anxious or have feelings of nothingness.*
☐ *Rather than looking forward to the future, you feel hopeless and/or pessimistic.*
☐ *You feel overwhelmed by feelings of guilt, worthlessness, and/or helplessness.*
☐ *You feel more irritable and restless, and the people you know start asking you why you are being cranky.*
☐ *You have no interest in doing things you enjoy, including sex.*
☐ *You are more tired than usual, and you feel fatigued.*
☐ *Your memory is not as good as it was, and you have difficulty concentrating, remembering details, and making decisions.*
☐ *There is a change in your sleeping pattern. You can't sleep, you are waking up in the early morning, or you are sleeping too much.*
☐ *Without trying, your weight has changed; you are eating less or more than usual.*
☐ *You have been thinking about ending all your problems by killing yourself.*
☐ *Even with treatment, you seem to have persistent aches or pains, headaches, cramps, or digestive problems.*

138

Now reread the list and mark the statements that describe what you have been feeling for at least two weeks. Did you check more than three of these statements? If you did, you should take this list to your health care provider and ask that person what you should do to get better.

Q *Can I get better?*
Yes. There are people who suffer with their depression and never seek professional help. To get better, however, most people need to seek professional help. A combination of medication and psychotherapy has been shown to have the best outcomes. New research also has pointed to the benefits of exercise to reduce depression, and there is increasing support for the use of light therapy to treat mood disorders. The important point is that you can get much better and enjoy life again.

Your health care provider should be able to direct you to a mental health professional for psychotherapy. Selecting a psychotherapist is a very personal decision. You need to find someone you feel comfortable with and someone you feel understands your experiences, community, and language.

Q *What if someone I know has depression?*
While being supportive of that person's struggles, you must also encourage her or him to seek professional help. If someone starts to talk about suicide, you must take that fact seriously and discuss it with anyone who is caring for that person, or you should call a hotline for guidance on what to do next. Be aware that people who hit bottom and are starting to get better are at an increased risk for suicide.

WHERE TO LEARN MORE

NATIONAL LIBRARY OF MEDICINE (NLM): MEDLINEPLUS
www.nlm.nih.gov/medlineplus/depression.html
The NLM is the library resource for NIH, and it provides depression-related news, overviews, and research findings, plus information about prevention, symptoms, alternative therapies, and clinical trials.

NATIONAL INSTITUTE FOR MENTAL HEALTH (NIMH)
www.nimh.nih.gov/health/topics/depression
The NIMH is part of the NIH, and its website describes the various forms of depression and provides information on the detection, treatment, and management of depression.

NATIONAL MENTAL HEALTH ASSOCIATION (NMHA)
www.depression-screening.org
The NMHA, a not-for-profit organization, offers a confidential depression screening test online. The site also provides information on symptoms, treatments, and ways to live with depression.

Diabetes

"Every person in my family has it."

LATINAS AND DIABETES

- *Among Hispanics twenty years or older, 10.4 percent have diabetes.*

- *Among Hispanics, the diabetes prevalence rates are 8.2 percent for Cubans, 11.9 percent for Mexican Americans, and 12.6 percent for Puerto Ricans.*

- *Women are more likely than men to have diabetes.*

- *Latinas have a higher rate of diabetes (111.8 individuals per 1,000 adults) than do non-Hispanic white women (69.4 individuals per 1,000 adults).*

- *Between ages forty-five and seventy-four, the prevalence of diabetes increases with age for most Americans.*

Q *Que pasa?*
Everyone's blood has to contain some glucose (sugar). In people who do not have diabetes, the normal range is about 70 to 120 mg/dl. Diabetes is the cluster of diseases defined by having a level of blood sugar (blood glucose) that is higher than what is good for you. There are three main types of diabetes, although recent research has suggested that more types of diabetes will be discovered.

Type 1, previously called juvenile diabetes or insulin-dependent diabetes, is usually diagnosed in children, teenagers, or young adults. Approximately 5 percent to 10 percent of people with diabetes have type 1. This type of diabetes is due to a malfunction of the immune system. For some reason a person's immune system, which usually protects the body, mistakenly attacks and destroys the cells in the pancreas that produce insulin. If you have type 1 diabetes, controlling its effects will likely mean taking insulin by injection or pump, making healthy eating choices, and having a regular exercise program. You will also need to control your blood pressure and keep your cholesterol at healthy levels. Some people with diabetes also will be encouraged to take an aspirin each day.

Type 2, formerly called adult-onset diabetes, occurs when the body either does not make enough insulin or cannot effectively use the insulin it makes. Approximately 90 percent to 95 percent of people with diabetes have type 2. Although it is usually found in people forty or older, type 2 diabetes may also be found in children and teens. Some people have no symptoms, and others develop symptoms gradually. The symptoms include feeling tired or ill; urinating frequently (especially at night); or having unusual thirst, weight loss, blurred vision, frequent infections, and slow-healing wounds.

Gestational diabetes occurs during pregnancy. Although this form of diabetes usually goes away after the baby is born, it is a strong indicator that the woman is much more likely to develop diabetes later in life. The estimate is that women who have gestational diabetes have a 20 percent to 50 percent chance of developing diabetes, mostly type 2, in the next five to ten years.

Prediabetes is the condition in which people have a level of blood glucose slightly lower than that among people with diabetes. People with prediabetes are at risk of developing type 2 diabetes. This condition is also sometimes called impaired glucose tolerance or impaired fasting glucose.

> **MYTH:** Latinas have the gene for diabetes.
> **FACT:** There is no single gene for diabetes, but there are clusters of genes that may put someone at risk of developing diabetes.
>
> ---
>
> **MYTH:** Since Latinas are likely to have diabetes and carry excess weight, we are more likely to have heart disease than are non-Hispanic white women.
> **FACT:** Latinas have less heart disease than non-Hispanic white women do, even though we are more likely to have diabetes and carry excess weight.

Diabetes that is not controlled can lead to serious problems with your heart, eyes, kidneys, nerves, gums, and teeth; it can also lead to death.

CAUSES AND PREVENTION

It is not known what causes type 1, type 2, or gestational diabetes. We do not know what the risk factors for type 1 diabetes are. We do know that there are many risk factors for getting type 2 diabetes and that you can take the following steps to decrease the chance of getting it or to delay the onset:

- *Reduce excess weight.*
- *Reduce high blood pressure.*
- *Reduce abnormal cholesterol (lipid) levels.*
- *Begin a regular exercise program.*

Here are the risk factors that you cannot change but that you need to consider:

- *Family history of diabetes*
- *Being forty-five or older*

- *History of diabetes while pregnant (gestational diabetes)*
- *History of polycystic ovarian syndrome (PCOS)*
- *History of blood vessel problems affecting the heart, brain, or legs*
- *History of dark, thick, and velvety patches of skin around the neck and armpits*

We also know that physical activity plays an important part in preventing type 2 diabetes. Research has shown that physical activity can improve the body's ability to use insulin. There has been some success with delaying or preventing the onset of type 2 diabetes for persons with prediabetes by having them lose 5 percent to 7 percent of their body weight, be physically active for thirty minutes on five days each week, and make healthy food choices.

Some risk factors for gestational diabetes include having a parent, brother, or sister with diabetes; being twenty-five or older; being overweight; having already had gestational diabetes; giving birth to at least one baby weighing more than nine pounds; or being diagnosed with prediabetes.

HEALTH POINT

Latinas have higher rates of gestational (pregnancy-related) diabetes than do non-Hispanic white women.

Q Do I have a problem?

The symptoms for type 1 diabetes usually develop over a short time and include increased thirst and urination, constant hunger, weight loss, blurred vision, and extreme fatigue.

Type 2 diabetes is usually found in people older than forty, but it may also be found in children and teens. Some people have no symptoms, and others develop symptoms gradually. The symptoms include feeling tired or ill; urinating frequently (especially at night); or having unusual thirst, weight loss, blurred vision, frequent infections, and slow-healing wounds.

Since we do not know what causes gestational diabetes, all women get screened as part of prenatal care. Latinas may be screened earlier because we are more likely to have this condition develop during pregnancy.

Q *Can I get better?*
Diabetes is a condition you can manage. Depending on the type of diabetes you have, your health care provider will give you specific instructions on what you can do to control your condition. You will most likely be asked to do the following:

- *Maintain a healthy eating plan*

- *Increase your physical activity*

- *Take your medicines as prescribed*

- *Monitor your blood glucose level as recommended*

- *Maintain your health journal*

- *Visit your health care provider on a regular basis and take other tests as needed. While you can measure your blood glucose level at home, you should also take your blood glucose (A1C) test twice a year when you visit your health care provider. This test looks at how you have been managing your blood glucose level over the past few months. In other words, the results reveal whether or not you have strayed from your target glucose level.*

The goal is to keep your blood glucose level as close as possible to the level of someone who does not have diabetes. The closer to normal you keep your level of blood glucose, the lower your chances are of developing serious health problems.

Q *What if someone I know has diabetes?*
What we, as Latinas, can give—which is more valuable than anything else—is support to someone who has diabetes. You can help by learning and sharing what you find out about diabetes, foods that are healthy to eat, different foods and recipes to try, and activities you can do together. Finding new ways to spend time together can be a huge boost, such as going for a walk rather than just sitting. In terms of food, you could join your family member or friend in switching from white bread to whole wheat bread.

Research has clearly shown that what is most reinforcing for Latinas is a sense of support that makes us feel we belong. It is more important than instrumental support, such as offering to give someone a ride. Use your strengths as a Latina to help the people you care about so that they can get better and manage their condition.

WHERE TO LEARN MORE

NATIONAL DIABETES INFORMATION CLEARINGHOUSE (NDIC)
diabetes.niddk.nih.gov
The NDIC provides educational materials to increase knowledge and understanding about diabetes among patients, health care professionals, and the general public.

NATIONAL LIBRARY OF MEDICINE (NLM): MEDLINEPLUS
www.nlm.nih.gov/medlineplus/diabetes.html
The NLM is the library resource for the NIH, and it offers links to news on diabetes, including general articles, treatments, specific conditions, prevention, management, and statistics.

National Diabetes Education Program (NDEP)

www.ndep.nih.gov

The NDEP, a partnership of the National Institutes of Health and the Centers for Disease Control and Prevention, provides information on diabetes prevention and treatment.

CDC Diabetes Program

www.cdc.gov/diabetes/

This CDC program provides information about common symptoms, risk factors, and management options for diabetes.

American Diabetes Association

www.diabetes.org/about-diabetes.jsp

This not-for-profit organization offers information on diabetes.

National Institute on Aging and NASA

weboflife.nasa.gov/exerciseandaging/cover.html

This animated guide is an excellent introduction to exercises for people forty-five or older.

Heart Attack

"It's nothing—I just need to rest a little."

LATINAS AND HEART ATTACKS

- *Latinas with symptoms of a heart attack delay significantly longer before going to a hospital than do non-Hispanic whites. (In the next section we look at more information on Latinas and heart disease.)*

Q *Que pasa?*
Your heart is not able to function.

Q *Do I have a problem?*
Here are the warning signs for a heart attack:

- *Your chest feels different, weird, or painful. You may feel like there is pressure on your chest, a squeezing feeling, a sense of fullness, or pain. These feelings may be mild to severe. They can also last a few minutes or come and go. It feels different than when you have muscle pain. While chest pain or discomfort is the most common symptom of heart attack, 43 percent of women do not experience it.*

- *You have an odd feeling or discomfort in your upper body. This could be in one or both arms, or in the back, neck, jaw, or stomach.*

- *You can take only short breaths. This may occur either before or after you feel the discomfort in your chest.*

- *You feel like vomiting or fainting. You may also break out in a cold sweat or feel lightheaded.*

> **MYTH:** When you have a heart attack, you just keel over and die.
>
> **FACT:** Ninety-five percent of women experience symptoms before having a heart attack.

Women experience more "atypical" symptoms at the time of a heart attack than men do. In one study, women were more than twice as likely as men to experience nausea, vomiting, or indigestion.

Not everyone having a heart attack experiences the same symptoms. Some will have all of these symptoms, while others will have one. Even if you have had one heart attack, the symptoms may not be the same if you have another.

Too often, Latinas who are experiencing a heart attack will wait longer than they should before going to the hospital. The longer you wait, the more damage there will be to your heart if you are having a heart attack. Every minute counts toward saving your heart. If you are having a heart attack, the faster you can get care and medication, the better the outcome will be for you.

HEALTH POINT

Call 911. Do not drive yourself to the hospital.

If you think you are having a heart attack, you need to call 911. In most places, ambulances have the staff and equipment to help stabilize you. For example, most ambulances bring oxygen and medications, including aspirin. You should not drive yourself to the hospital.

Q *Can I get better?*
Yes. Your health care provider will talk to you about what to do to stay well and will help you plan out the changes you need to make in your life.

WHERE TO LEARN MORE

NATIONAL HEART, LUNG, AND BLOOD INSTITUTE (NHLBI)
www.nhlbi.nih.gov
The NHLBI is the primary part of the National Institutes of Health. doing research on heart and vascular diseases.

NATIONAL LIBRARY OF MEDICINE (NLM): MEDLINEPLUS
www.nlm.nih.gov/medlineplus/heartdiseaseinwomen.html
The NLM is the library resource for the NIH, and it has extensive information on women and heart disease.

CDC—HEART DISEASE HOME
www.cdc.gov/heartdisease
Heart disease is the leading cause of death in the United States and a focus of the work of the CDC.

OFFICE ON WOMEN'S HEALTH
www.4woman.gov/faq/heart-disease
The website of this federal office answers many questions, such as the following: What does high cholesterol have to do with heart disease? Does using the birth control patch increase my risk for heart disease?

AMERICAN COLLEGE OF CARDIOLOGY
www.cardiosmart.org
Cardiosmart is a consumer information service of the American College of Cardiology Foundation. Under "Learn About Your Heart Disease" consumer information is available in English and selected topics in Spanish.

AMERICAN HEART ASSOCIATION
www.americanheart.org
This national not-for profit organization seeks to reduce disability and death from cardiovascular diseases and stroke and offers extensive information for consumers.

Heart Disease

"Me duele el corazón." (My heart hurts.)

LATINAS AND HEART DISEASE

- *Heart disease is the number one killer of Latinas.*
- *Latinas are less like to have heart disease than non-Hispanic white women are.*
- *Latinas with symptoms of a heart attack delay significantly longer before going to a hospital than do non-Hispanic whites.*

Q *Que pasa?*
Your heart is at the core of a system of blood vessels and electrical impulses that make it possible for blood to be pumped to every part of your body. Much of what we know about heart disease is based on decades of research on men, but recent research has begun identifying the unique aspects of the female heart. At a structural level, we know that the blood vessels surrounding a woman's heart are smaller than those surrounding a man's. In a presentation to an audience in New York, the renowned cardiologist Dr. Mehmet Oz (of Columbia University) described a woman's heart-surrounding blood vessels as being like capellini (*fideo,* or angel hair pasta) and a man's being like linguine. These differences are important when the treatment recommendation is surgery or other invasive procedures.

Cardiovascular disease includes the many possible conditions that prevent your heart from doing its job properly. These diseases may be due to several malfunctions:

- *The blood vessels are clogged or blocked, making it harder for your heart to work. If they are too clogged, your heart will stop working (coronary artery disease).*

- *The electrical impulses that help your heart pump are not working well (arrhythmias).*

- *Parts of the heart itself (e.g., chambers, valves) are not working well.*

- *In addition, some people are born with problems in their heart. These are called congenital heart problems.*

CAUSES AND PREVENTION

There is no single cause for heart disease. There are many things you can do to decrease the likelihood that you will get heart disease:

- *Avoid all tobacco smoke—first-, second-, and thirdhand smoke.*

- *Restrict your outdoor activity when the air quality is not good. Do this even though the warnings focus on children, older persons, and persons with respiratory problems.*

- *Focus on getting fit and making movement part of your life.*

- *Think about what you are eating and the impact it will have on your heart and cells.*

- *Maintain a healthy weight.*

- *Prevent or control high blood pressure, diabetes, high cholesterol, and high triglycerides. If you are taking medicines, be sure that you take them as directed by your health care provider.*

- *If you drink alcohol, you may want to consider having one glass of red wine a day (five ounces) since research has shown*

MYTH:	If I have bad teeth, my heart will have problems, too.
FACT:	Inflammation of your gums does not cause inflammation of your arteries. It just means that something is causing an inflammatory response by your body. Inflammation is the body's response to injury or infection.

MYTH:	Only people with high cholesterol have to worry about heart attacks.
FACT:	Half of all people who have heart attacks have normal cholesterol levels.

that this may be good for the heart. Skipping a few days, though, does not mean that you can make up for the days you missed by drinking more on one day. Heavy drinking can damage the heart muscle and worsen other risk factors for heart disease.

- *If your breathing stops or gets very shallow while you are sleeping, you may have sleep apnea. You need to talk to your health care provider about this, since sleep apnea raises your risk of having heart disease.*

- *Avoid some of the common triggers for heart attacks, such as emotionally upsetting events (particularly ones in which you experience anger) or overexertion.*

- *Women who use birth control pills or use the birth control patch need to consider whether or not they may be at an increased risk for heart disease. This is particularly true for women over thirty-five and for all women who smoke.*

- *Reconsider the risks and benefits of menopausal hormone therapy (MHT) by talking through the issues with your health care provider.*

HEALTH POINT

Because your heart and lungs work together, being near tobacco smoke is bad for your heart.

What many Latinas fear most is having a heart attack. It is important to remember that a heart attack is not a disease but a huge sign that your heart is not able to work. A heart attack may be the result of any of the cardiovascular conditions just discussed.

Q *Do I have a problem? Now what?*
Heart disease often has no symptoms; even women with a healthy weight who are fit may have heart disease. Your regular wellness visit will help your health care provider determine whether you need further testing and treatment. Depending on your risk factors, your visit may include:

- *Electrocardiogram (ECG or EKG). This test measures the electrical activity of the heart as it contracts and relaxes. The electrical pattern is recorded on a graph. By reading the ECG, your health care provider will be able to see how your heart is working.*

- *Blood tests. Some tests identify enzymes or other substances that are released when cells begin to die.*

After reviewing your test results, your health care provider may suggest that you schedule a visit with a cardiologist (a health care provider who specializes in cardiovascular disease) and go for additional tests. A treadmill test is often used as a screening tool for diagnosing heart disease. This test, however, has proven less effective in diagnosing problems and disease in women than in men. In a recent study, the results from the treadmill test were incorrect for more than a third of the women studied. Before scheduling a treadmill test, you should talk with your health care provider about the value of this test and about other possible tests.

In the meantime, to keep our heart healthy we have to try to manage the risk factors that are under our control. There is increasing evidence that inflammation plays a major role in heart disease. Research is under way to understand and control the inflammatory process.

We are learning more about the female heart every day.

Q *Can I get better?*
Most definitely. Not only can you get better, but once your heart is working well, you will also feel better. There have been major advances in the treatment of heart disease through the use of medication and the control of risk factors. There was a time when the only treatment available was major surgery or a heart transplant. Now there are many options.

Q *What if someone I know has heart disease?*
Using the risk factors just discussed as a starting point, you can help create a sense of community that makes it easy for your family member or friend to take the necessary steps toward having a healthy heart. Making sure that it is easy to eat healthy foods at home, avoiding smoke, getting fit, and taking medicines as directed are good steps for everyone's health. You can support others by helping them make regular wellness visits and keep their "About My Health" tools up to date.

Where to learn more

National Library of Medicine (NLM): MedlinePlus
www.nlm.nih.gov/medlineplus/heartdiseaseinwomen.html
The NLM is the library resource for NIH and has up-to-date information for consumers.

National Heart, Lung, and Blood Institute (NHLBI)
www.nhlbi.nih.gov
The NHLBI is the primary part of the National Institutes of Health. doing research on heart and vascular diseases.

Office on Women's Health
www.4woman.gov/faq/heart-disease.

CDC—Heart Disease Home
www.cdc.gov/heartdisease

American College of Cardiology
www.cardiosmart.org
Cardiosmart is a consumer information service of the American College of Cardiology Foundation. Under "Learn About Your Heart Disease" consumer information is available in English and selected topics in Spanish.

American Heart Association
www.americanheart.org
This national not-for profit organization seeks to reduce disability and death from cardiovascular diseases and stroke.

Women's Heart Foundation
www.womensheart.org
This nonprofit foundation is dedicated to the care and treatment of women's hearts.

High Blood Pressure (Hypertension)

"I feel fine, so I know my blood pressure is normal."

LATINAS AND HIGH BLOOD PRESSURE

- *Latinas are less likely to know that they have high blood pressure.*

Q *Que pasa?*
Your heart exerts pressure against the walls of your blood vessels when it beats (systolic pressure) and when it is at rest (diastolic pressure). That is why your blood pressure is said as two numbers, for instance 110 over 80. The first number is the systolic pressure, and the second is the diastolic pressure.

The following chart shows what your blood pressure reading means:

CATEGORY	SYSTOLIC		DIASTOLIC
Low	Less than 90	or	Less than 60
Normal	Less than 120	and	Less than 80
Pre-hypertension	120–139	or	80–89
Stage I hypertension	140–159	or	90–99
Stage II hypertension	160 or higher	or	100 or higher

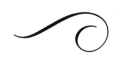

> **MYTH:** You can always tell when your blood pressure is high.
> **FACT:** In most cases there are no symptoms at all.
>
> ---
>
> **MYTH:** Only Latinas who are overweight have to worry about high blood pressure (hypertension).
> **FACT:** Latinas who have healthy weights may have high blood pressure.

It is important for all of us—and especially for pregnant women—to know what our blood pressure is. Since high blood pressure very often has no symptoms, you need to have your blood pressure checked on a regular basis.

Uncontrolled hypertension may lead to stroke, heart disease, visual abnormalities, kidney failure, and hardening of the arteries (arteriosclerosis). High blood pressure that develops during pregnancy may be a serious condition requiring close monitoring by your health care provider.

CAUSES AND PREVENTION

For 95 percent of the people who have hypertension, we do not know the cause, so their hypertension is called essential or primary. The other 5 percent have secondary hypertension, which is caused by some other condition such as diabetes or kidney failure.

By taking the following familiar healthy actions, you can reduce the chances of having high blood pressure: do not smoke, maintain a healthy weight, engage in physical activity on a regular basis, reduce sodium in what you eat and drink to 1,500 milligrams (mg) of sodium (in other words, two-thirds of a teaspoon of salt) per day, do not drink alcohol in excess (more than one drink a day for women), and try to reduce (not just manage) stress in your life.

Q *Can I get better?*
While there is no cure for hypertension, there is much you can do to manage and control your blood pressure. If you have high blood pressure, you need to very carefully and consistently follow the treatment plan developed by your health care provider. While sometimes changes in your eating patterns, your activity level, and other lifestyle factors can help you control your high blood pressure, such steps may not be enough and you may need to take medication.

If you take medicine, you have to remember to take it as your health care provider explained to do. This is especially true on those days when you are feeling well. Remember that if you are feeling fine, it is because the medicine is working and you need to continue taking it. As with any other medication, do not stop taking your medication without discussing such a step with your health care provider. To control your blood pressure on a regular basis, your health care provider will encourage you to measure it and keep a written record of your readings. You may choose to buy a blood pressure monitor to take your blood pressure at home or you may take it at the free blood pressure monitors available in some stores.

HEALTH POINT

Sazón that is prepackaged may be mostly salt or sodium; read the food label to know what you are eating.

Q *What if someone I know has high blood pressure?*
There is much you can do to support those you know who have high blood pressure. To begin with, you can help them maintain healthy habits with respect to what and how they eat. Removing the salt shaker from the table is a simple way to start, and encouraging walks after a meal is also a good idea for everybody.

Where to learn more

National Library of Medicine (NLM): MedlinePlus
www.nlm.nih.gov/medlineplus/tutorials/hypertension/
htm/index.htm

National Heart, Lung, and Blood Institute (NHLBI)
www.nhlbi.nih.gov

American College of Cardiology
www.cardiosmart.org

American Heart Association
www.americanheart.org

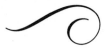

HIV/AIDS

"I had no idea my husband was HIV positive."

LATINAS AND HIV/AIDS

• *Latinas are four times more likely to be HIV positive than non-Hispanic white women are.*

In 2006 there were 20,004 cases of Latinas living with HIV/AIDS.

• *Latinas are less likely to use a condom than are other women.*

Q *Que pasa?*
When you are exposed to the human immunodeficiency virus (HIV), it can be in your body for more than twenty years before you develop the acquired immunodeficiency syndrome (AIDS). You can get the virus through sexual contact and blood-to-blood transfer.

A woman who is HIV positive can pass the virus to her baby throughout her pregnancy, during childbirth, and during breastfeeding. On the positive side, newborns who are properly treated now have a very high likelihood of not developing HIV and women who do have HIV can live healthy lives for many years when undergoing treatments based on the latest recommendations.

CAUSES AND PREVENTION

HIV/AIDS has been part of our public discussion for nearly thirty years. And yet in 2006, when the CDC reported the data on new AIDS cases among adolescent and adult females,

> **MYTH:** You have to have anal intercourse to be at risk.
>
> **FACT:** Women who have oral or vaginal intercourse are also at risk.
>
> ———————————————
>
> **MYTH:** If you are HIV positive, there is nothing you can do to deal with the health-related effects.
>
> **FACT:** If you are HIV positive, you should start taking medications as soon as possible.

Latinas had the highest rates of high-risk heterosexual contact. As Latinas, we need to take care of ourselves and be honest about our relationships.

There is no cure for HIV/AIDS, only treatment. The possibility of a vaccine seems fairly distant. To protect yourself you can choose which actions you will take:

- *Abstain from oral, anal, and vaginal sex.*

- *Choose a monogamous relationship with someone who has tested HIV negative. This action assumes that both you and your partner will remain monogamous.*

- *Do not share needles if you use drugs.*

- *Use condoms. (According to the NIAID, male latex condoms or female polyurethane condoms may offer partial protection during oral, anal, or vaginal sex. Only water-based lubricants should be used with male latex condoms.*

Q *Do I have a problem?*
Do you think you have been exposed to the virus? It takes six weeks to a year for your body to develop blood levels of the virus that can be detected. It is important to know your HIV status and the status of your partner, and

there are many ways to get this crucial information. You can buy a home test kit or go to one of the many free testing sites (call 1-866-783-2645 for locations).

Most people who get infected will have no symptoms. Some may get what feels like the flu (fever, headache, tiredness, enlarged lymph nodes in the neck and groin) within a month or two after exposure to the virus. During this time people are very infectious, and HIV is present in large quantities in genital fluids. But for most people there are no symptoms for ten or more years. Although they may feel fine, the virus is in their body and working to kill off the immune system. Other symptoms that may appear before the onset of AIDS include lack of energy; weight loss; frequent fevers and sweats; persistent or frequent yeast infections (oral or vaginal); persistent skin rashes or flaky skin; pelvic inflammatory disease that does not respond to treatment; short-term memory loss; and frequent and severe herpes infections that cause shingles or mouth, genital, or anal sores.

HEALTH POINT

For important information about other serious and all-too-common STDs, see the upcoming "Sexually Transmitted Diseases" discussion.

Q Can I get better?
Although there is no cure for HIV/AIDS, you can live a full life. With the treatment advances we have experienced, HIV/AIDS is becoming a chronic disease. With early identification and medication, many people with HIV are living longer and having a normal life expectancy.

Q What if someone I know has HIV/AIDS?
You should treat the person as you usually would. If this is someone with whom you are sexually intimate, you have to discuss what precautions you both will take so that you will not get the virus. You may also want to make sure that this person's health care provider is someone who

specializes in HIV/AIDS treatment. If someone in your household is HIV positive, you have to take precautions to ensure that there is no contact between your skin or mucous membranes and the person's blood. According to the CDC, here are some prudent steps to take:

- *Wear plastic or rubber gloves during contact with blood or other body fluids that could contain visible blood, such as urine, feces, or vomit.*

- *Use bandages to cover any skin exposed by cuts, sores, or breaks, whether on you or the person who is HIV positive.*

- *Immediately wash hands and other parts of the body that may have had contact with blood or other body fluids. Appropriately disinfect any surfaces that have been soiled with blood.*

- *Avoid practices that increase the likelihood of blood contact, such as sharing razors and toothbrushes.*

- *Use needles and other sharp instruments only when medically necessary, and handle them according to recommendations for health-care settings. (Do not put caps back on needles by hand or remove needles from syringes. Dispose of needles in puncture-proof containers out of the reach of children and visitors.)*

WHERE TO LEARN MORE

NATIONAL LIBRARY OF MEDICINE (NLM): MedlinePlus
www.nlm.nih.gov/medlineplus/aids.htm
The NLM is the library resource for the NIH, and it provides links to news and articles on AIDS and HIV infection. Also, the NLM covers information on the disease's prevention, its symptoms and treatment, clinical trials, and related research and statistics.

NATIONAL INSTITUTE ON ALLERGIES AND INFECTIOUS DISEASES (NIAID)
www.niaid.nih.gov
The NIAID, part of the NIH, is the premier research center on AIDS and other infectious diseases.

CDC—HIV/AIDS
www.cdc.gov/hiv
The CDC offers HIV/AIDS recommendations and guidelines, plus up-to-date information about the disease.

Immune System

"Where is it located? I'm not too certain what that is."

LATINAS AND THE IMMUNE SYSTEM

- *Latinas are more likely to have autoimmune disorders than non-Hispanic white women are.*

Q *Que pasa?*
The immune system is your bodyguard at the cellular level. It protects the cells that are "you" and isolates and destroys foreign materials. Bacteria, viruses, parasites, fungi—all those tiny microbes that we do not see but that are all around us—are put through a "security clearance" process by our immune system.

As you would expect, these security clearance areas are located throughout the body in different places: the tonsils and adenoids, the lymph nodes in the throat and the attached lymphatic vessels, the thymus (which is in the middle of the chest), the lymph nodes in armpits, the spleen (located on the body's left side, just about where the elbow touches), the appendix (on the body's right side, halfway between the elbow and wrist), Peyer's patch (to the left of the belly button), lymph nodes and lymphatic vessels in the inner leg area, and the bone marrow throughout the body. All of these sites have small white blood cells (lymphocytes) that use the blood vessels and lymphatic vessels to travel throughout the body and screen any incoming microbes.

The system works to produce a variety of cells that destroy, penetrate, or attack other cells. Sometimes you can acquire immunity to a condition, because once the immune system has successfully attacked an invader, it retains knowledge of

> **MYTH:** Your appendix, spleen, and tonsils are useless.
> **FACT:** These organs are part of your immune system.
>
> **MYTH:** Hormones have no effect on the immune system.
> **FACT:** Hormones and tiny networks of fibers communicate from the brain to the cells of the immune system.

what the system did. The next time an invasion is launched, the system can respond swiftly and even more effectively. You get this immunity from your own exposures (this includes vaccines) and from what you inherit.

The problem is that in some cases the microbes are able to adapt and get in the body by using a different strategy. At other times the cells mistake your own cells for being foreign and responds by creating cells to attack them.

When your immune system is working to defend you from microbes, what you experience is not comfortable sometimes, but it is your body trying to fight off the enemy. For example, fever, coughs, and sneezes are very important to your health. A fever kills off the many microbes that cannot survive in temperatures higher than 98.6, such as flu viruses. When your body produces mucus, it creates a medium for getting germs out of your body, so coughs and sneezes can help with that process. Other strategies that your immune system uses include inflammation, vomiting, diarrhea, fatigue, and cramping.

As of now, there were few diagnostic tests available to detect specific immune-system problems. Only now are we beginning to understand how the immune system works and what different diseases can develop when it does not work well.

CAUSES AND PREVENTION
Disorders of the immune system result because the system is doing either less or more than it should.

Less. *Immunodeficiency* means that the immune system is not very active and does not protect you. This can be due to an inherited disorder, an infection, or medication. Temporary suppression of your immune system can be due to blood transfusions, surgery, malnutrition, smoking, or stress.

Too much. When your immune system is more active than it should be, it begins to attack you. The diseases that result are called autoimmune diseases, and the most familiar ones are rheumatoid arthritis, type 1 diabetes, and lupus. If your immune system attacks harmless substances like pollen, then you have an allergy.

No one knows for certain what causes autoimmune diseases.

HEALTH POINT

The immune system is impacted by your feelings and the stress in your life.

THE FUTURE

Evidence is growing that will help us decipher the tremendous role that the immune system has in our health. New medicines are being developed to stimulate the immune system to defend the body. Additionally, the nature of wellness is changing as we find out more about what causes this system to work or to malfunction. Growing information about the contribution of our emotions to our health, for instance, will play an increasingly important role in understanding our immune system.

WHERE TO LEARN MORE

NATIONAL INSTITUTE ON ALLERGIES AND INFECTIOUS DISEASES (NIAID)
www.niaid.nih.gov
The NIAID, a part of the NIH, is the premier research center on AIDS and other infectious diseases.

Liver Disease

"Me duele mi hígado!" (My liver hurts!)

LATINAS AND LIVER DISEASE

- *Hispanics are the group most likely to be discharged from a hospital with a diagnosis of alcohol-related liver disease.*

- *Latinas have a higher incidence of liver cancer than do non-Hispanic white women.*

Q *Que pasa?*
If you understand Spanish, you may hear someone complain of having a liver that hurts or of feeling so annoyed that her or his bile is getting all stirred up. This is not something you would say in English. Perhaps this difference in what we say is based in the reality that Hispanics are more likely to get liver disease than non-Hispanics are.

The liver is your biggest organ. That is very good because it has to cleanse your blood of toxins, make protein, fight infections, produce bile to help digest food, and even store energy. It does a lot of work to keep you healthy.

When you have liver disease, the liver cannot do its many tasks. Diseases of the liver are also called hepatic diseases. Hepatitis is inflammation of the liver, and it can be due to scarring that has occurred from damage or injury (e.g., cirrhosis, fatty liver disease), viruses (hepatitis A, B, or C), cancer (hepatocellular carcinoma), or problems with the immune system (type 1 and type 2 autoimmune hepatitis). Hemochromatosis is another liver disease, but it is rare and inherited.

169

MYTH: Liver disease is not a problem for Hispanics.
FACT: Hispanics are more likely to die from liver disease than non-Hispanic whites are.

MYTH: Whenever you feel sick, you should take an antibiotic.
FACT: Antibiotics are the greatest cause of drug-induced liver damage.

Using drugs, being exposed to toxins, or drinking too much alcohol can scar your liver. Once you have scar tissue in your liver, it will not go away. If there is too much scarring and your liver cannot work properly, the only option left may be a liver transplant.

CAUSES AND PREVENTION

Drinking too much alcohol, abusing medications, and being exposed to toxic chemicals in the water you drink or food you eat can lead to cirrhosis, which scars the liver. Viruses also cause liver diseases. Each kind of hepatitis virus (viral hepatitis) is spread in a specific way.

Hepatitis A (HAV) is spread primarily through food or water contaminated by coming into contact with even microscopic pieces of feces from someone who has HAV. You can be exposed to HAV through contact with someone who is infected and did not wash her or his hands thoroughly after going to the bathroom or contact with water that has been contaminated by the feces of someone who has HAV. You also can be exposed to HAV by having oral or anal sex with someone who has HAV.

Hepatitis B (HBV) is spread through contact with blood, semen, or other body fluid from someone who has HBV. A woman with HBV can pass the virus to her baby at birth.

Hepatitis C (HCV) is spread through contact with the blood of a person who has it. Whether a person has had such contact is sometimes difficult to know, since most people who are infected with HCV do not have any symptoms for years.

A woman with HBV or HCV can pass the virus to her baby at birth. There are vaccines only for HAV and HBV. A blood test can show whether you have HBV or HCV.

There is no known cause for either type 1 or type 2 autoimmune hepatitis. Type 1 starts in teenagers or young adults, with half of the people also having another autoimmune disease. Type 2 is usually found in girls aged two to fourteen, and it is much less common.

Q *Do I have a problem?*
Sometimes it is hard to tell whether you have hepatitis, since some people do not have symptoms. People with HAV and HBV usually do not have symptoms. When there are symptoms, these may include loss of appetite, nausea and vomiting, diarrhea, dark-colored urine, pale bowel movements, stomach pain, and yellowing of the skin and eyes (jaundice).

As mentioned earlier, there is a blood test for HBV and HCV. A liver biopsy is sometimes used to make a diagnosis of liver disease.

Q *Can I get better?*
Although HAV and HBV both cause inflammation of the liver, they also tend to get better on their own after several weeks (HAV) or months (HBV). If HBV does not get better, it is called chronic HBV, which can lead to cirrhosis or liver cancer. HCV does not get better by itself, and even with treatment the infection can last a lifetime.

HEALTH POINT

Antiobiotics are strong medicine and should be used only as direceted by your health care provider.

Q What if someone I know has liver disease?
The steps you take will depend on what type of liver disease the person has. Since alcohol will further damage the liver, you should do everything you can to help the person stop consuming alcohol and avoid exposure to toxic substances. If the person has HBC or HCV, you should reduce your exposure to her or his blood, semen, or other body fluids. For everyone, thoroughly washing hands after going to the bathroom or changing diapers or before preparing food is also a good practice to follow. This means spending at least twenty seconds washing your hands with soap and running water.

WHERE TO LEARN MORE

NATIONAL INSTITUTE OF DIABETES AND DIGESTIVE DISEASES, AND KIDNEY DISEASES (NIDDK)
www.niddk.nih.gov
The NIDDK is part of the NIH, and it is implementing the trans-NIH Action Plan for Liver Disease Research.

LATINO ORGANIZATION FOR LIVER AWARENESS (LOLA)
www.lola-national.org
This bilingual, bicultural organization is dedicated to raising awareness on liver disease through informational materials.

AMERICAN ASSOCIATION FOR THE STUDY OF LIVER DISEASES
www.aasld.org

AMERICAN LIVER FOUNDATION
www.liverfoundation.org

Lupus

"There's nothing wrong with her; she looks fine."

LATINAS AND LUPUS

- *Latinas are more likely to get lupus than are non-Hispanic white women.*

- *Latinas tend to develop symptoms at an earlier age than other women do.*

Q *Que pasa?*
Lupus develops when your immune system is out of balance, which causes it to become destructive to any organ or tissue in your body. An estimated 1.5 million people have a form of lupus.

- *Systemic lupus erythematosus (SLE) is the most common and most serious form of lupus. When you have systemic lupus, your immune system may cause inflammation in your joints, skin, kidneys, lungs, heart, blood vessels, nervous system, blood, and brain.*

- *Cutaneous lupus erythematosus is a form of lupus that affects only the skin. Cutaneous lupus causes rashes or sores (lesions), hair loss, and sores in the mouth and nose. The rashes usually appear on sun-exposed areas of the skin. One type of lesion is called a discoid lesion because it is shaped like a coin, or disk. Sometimes the lesions will cause scarring after they heal.*

- *Drug-induced lupus is a reaction to some prescription medicines. Symptoms include joint pain, skin rash, fever, and chest pain. When the medication is stopped, the symptoms will generally go away.*

- *Neonatal lupus is a rare form of lupus found in the newborn of a woman with lupus. Usually the symptoms are mild and disappear after the baby is six months old. Rarely, the baby's heart can be damaged, but this problem can be treated.*

CAUSES AND PREVENTION

We do not know what causes lupus; multiple factors such as hormones, genetics (heredity), and environment are all involved. We do know that lupus is not contagious—that is, you cannot "catch" lupus from someone or "give" lupus to anyone.

HEALTH POINT

Lupus is a difficult disease to diagnose, but once diagnosed there is much that you can do to control it.

Q How would I know if I have lupus?
The common symptoms of lupus—joint pain or swelling, muscle pain, extreme fatigue, fever with no known cause—are common to many other illnesses. Lupus symptoms also can come and go, and they can change over time. These are some of the reasons that lupus can be hard to diagnose.

Your health care provider may not know right away if you have lupus. A lupus diagnosis is made after careful review of your medical history, your symptoms, your laboratory test results, and the medical history of your close family members. Your health care provider may also need to look at a tiny piece of tissue taken from your skin or kidney (called a biopsy) before deciding whether you have lupus.

Q I have lupus. Now what?
People with lupus are generally treated by a rheumatologist, a physician who specializes in diseases of the joints and muscles. Depending on the type of lupus you have and your needs, other specialists will be consulted, such as a dermatologist for skin disease, a cardiologist for heart disease, or a nephrologist for kidney disease.

> **MYTH:** Lupus is found mostly in men.
> **FACT:** Nine out of ten people with lupus are women. Lupus can also occur in men, children, and teens.
>
> ---
>
> **MYTH:** You do not get lupus until you are older.
> **FACT:** Lupus develops most often between the ages of fifteen and forty-four, but it can occur at any age.
>
> ---
>
> **MYTH:** You will die from lupus within five years of its start.
> **FACT:** With proper treatment and care, most people with lupus will live a normal lifespan.

It is especially important to take a team approach to your health care when you have lupus. Together with your health care providers, you will develop a treatment plan to reduce swelling and pain in joints, prevent or reduce lupus flares, and prevent organ and tissue damage. You will learn ways to make your home and workplace more comfortable and less stressful. It is also very important to talk to your health care provider if you are planning to get pregnant, as an obstetrician who specializes in high-risk pregnancies should be added to your team.

Q Can I get better?

Although there is no cure for lupus, you can feel better. The earlier you get an accurate diagnosis and begin to receive treatment, the better your long-term health will be. Regular health care provider visits, keeping to your treatment plan, and lifestyle changes will minimize symptoms and improve your health over time. You can have the most up-to-date information by becoming active in the Lupus Foundation of America, Inc.

Q What if someone I know has lupus?
Help your friend or loved one create a healthy set of activities that you can enjoy together. Remember that the sun can cause disease flares. Be aware that lupus causes extreme fatigue, and sometimes your plans may have to be postponed. Learn to be a good listener.

WHERE TO LEARN MORE

NATIONAL INSTITUTE OF ARTHRITIS AND MUSCULOSKELETAL AND SKIN DISEASES (NIAMS)
www.niams.nih.gov/
The NIAMS, part of the National Institutes of Health (NIH), is the premier center for research on lupus.

LUPUS FOUNDATION OF AMERICA, INC.
www.lupus.org
The LFA is the foremost national nonprofit voluntary health organization dedicated to finding the causes of and cure for lupus, as well as providing support, services, and hope to all people affected by lupus. The LFA has a nationwide network of nearly three hundred chapters and support groups and operates programs of research, education, and advocacy.

AMERICAN COLLEGE OF RHEUMATOLOGY
www.rheumatology.org
This is the professional organization for rheumatology health care providers, scientists, researchers, and other health care professionals and the Association of Rheumatology Health Professionals, nonphysician health care professionals specializing in rheumatology, such as nurses, occupational therapists, physical therapists, psychologists, social workers, physician assistants, and educators. There is patient information in English and Spanish, as well as a listing of providers by location.

Menopause

"Tengo mucho calor!" (I am so hot!)

LATINAS AND MENOPAUSE

- *Latinas and non-Hispanic white women were equally likely to have hot flashes and night sweats.*

- *Latinas are significantly more likely than non-Hispanic white women to note mood changes, a decrease in energy, palpitations, breast tenderness, and memory loss.*

- *Latinas are less likely than non-Hispanic white women to report vaginal dryness.*

Q *Que pasa?*
Menopause is when a woman has not had a period for one year. At this point in life, a woman can no longer become pregnant, since her ovaries have stopped producing the hormones estrogen and progesterone. This usually occurs naturally and most often after age forty-five. These changes can occur over several years, and they may include a variety of other changes, too, such as the following:

- *Your period is no longer predictable in terms of the timing of when it will occur, how long it will fast, or how heavy or light it will be.*

- *You suddenly feel very warm and become uncomfortable because of hot flashes (which one of my amigas calls power surges).*

- *At night you may find that you get so hot that you sweat a lot, and then you get cold and feel chilly, which means you are experiencing night sweats.*

- *You have difficulty sleeping all through the night without waking up.*

- *Your vagina does not get as moist or wet as it did before; sometimes it feels dry.*

- *Your moods change or become changeable. Sometimes you seem to go from one extreme to another—sometimes you are cranky, and at other times you feel weepy.*

- *You seem more forgetful than usual.*

- *The hair on your head is falling out and getting thin, but you seem to have more hair growing on your face.*

Some women go through menopause before the age of forty. This is called premature ovarian failure, regardless of the reason. Usually, there is no explanation for why some of us go through menopause at a younger age; others of us may have had both ovaries removed, resulting in surgical menopause. If you do experience menopause before age forty, you should talk with your health care provider, since special testing may be able to determine the exact cause.

Postmenopause involves the years after menopause, and it begins after you go twelve months in a row without a period. This time—namely, the rest of your life—can be very happy and full.

Even though each one of us experiences menopause in her own unique way, it is good to talk to our *amigas* about their experiences and what they did and are doing. Maybe the fans that ladies used to carry in their purses are a good cultural tradition to embrace.

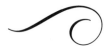

> **MYTH:** When you pass through menopause, you will no longer feel like a woman.
>
> **FACT:** Menstruation does not define a woman.
>
> ---
>
> **MYTH:** Latinas do not want to use menopausal hormone therapy.
>
> **FACT:** For unknown reasons, Latinas are more likely to use menopausal hormone therapy than are other women.

CAUSES AND PREVENTION

The cause of menopause is that you have lived long enough to get to that point in adulthood. There is no way to prevent menopause, as it is part of normal and healthy development. In the 1960s there was a movement to prevent menopause by keeping women artificially on estrogen. We now know that there are some increased risks for some cancers in doing that.

Q *Am I going through menopause? Now what?*
There are tests that may help to determine whether or not you are going through menopause. In addition, certain tests can be used to evaluate you for other conditions that may mimic menopause, such as an underactive thyroid gland. If you are experiencing some of the changes previously listed, you need to discuss them with your health care provider. Let your health care provider tell you whether or not you are going through menopause. Some of the changes that women experience during menopause can have other causes, and they may also be symptoms of more serious conditions.

To minimize the symptoms of menopause, you should focus on eating healthily and getting fit. Most women get through this time by making only slight adjustments in their daily routine. Surprisingly, more often than other women, Latinas get menopausal hormone therapy (MHT, formerly known as hormone replacement therapy or HRT). You should discuss with your health care provider the benefits and risks involved with this kind of treatment. If used for a limited time and for very specific reasons, menopausal hormone therapy (MHT) can relieve some of the moderate to severe menopausal symptoms. For some women, however, MHT may increase their chance of blood clots, heart attack, stroke, breast cancer, and gall bladder disease. If you decide to try MHT, use the lowest dose that helps for the shortest time you need it. Bioidentical hormone replacement therapy (BHRT) is another kind of artificial hormone, except these compounds are custom-made from a health care provider's prescription. These can be expensive, and your use of them needs to be very closely monitored.

Most "natural" treatments available for menopause are usually classified as supplements. Supplements have a much lower standard to meet in terms of safety, effectiveness, and reliability of ingredients in order to get approval from the Food and Drug Administration. Supplements include phytoestrogens (estrogen-like substances from a plant) that are found in soy and herbs such as black cohosh, wild yam, dong quai, and valerian root. According to the Office on Women's Health in the U.S. Department of Health and Human Services, there is no proof that these herbs (or pills or creams containing these herbs) help with hot flashes.

Here are some of the most common experiences women have had with menopause and some of the lessons on how to reduce their impact on your activities:

HEALTH POINT

Menopause is a healthy part of our life. However, if you are having symptoms that are affecting your ability to enjoy life—such as chronic lack of sleep, irritability, or extreme hot flashes—there are simple treatments that may be worth trying.

- **HOT FLASHES.** *The best thing to do is wear layers of clothing so that you can take off and put back on the different layers as your temperature fluctuates. You may also want to keep a more detailed entry in your "About My Health" tool (included in Part Three) to see if there is a pattern of what triggers your flashes.*

- **YOUR VAGINA DOES NOT GET LUBRICATED LIKE IT DID BEFORE.** *First, make certain that nothing has changed with how you feel about your partner or how your partner feels about you and that you still want sexual intimacy. If all those are still the same and you find that you are not as moist as you need to be, there are products you can buy to make intercourse pleasurable for both of you. A water-based, over-the-counter vaginal lubricant or vaginal moisturizer can be purchased without a prescription. Do not use petroleum jelly. If you continue to have this concern, your health care provider may prescribe a vaginal estrogen product in the form of creams, tablets, or a vaginal ring.*

- **YOU CANNOT SLEEP THROUGH THE NIGHT.** *Try to create a sleep sanctuary for yourself. If at all possible, keep your bedroom or sleeping area only for sleeping or for sexual intimacy. Try to develop a sleep routine that involves a series of steps to get you in the mindset for sleep. For example, kiss everyone good night, pick out your clothes for the next day, take a shower or bath, brush your hair, brush your teeth, get into bed, and say your prayers or think other calming thoughts. Keep your room as dark and quiet as possible. Try to keep your mind on peaceful images and thoughts.*

- **YOUR MOOD GOES FROM ONE EXTREME TO ANOTHER.** *To stabilize your moods, try to get regular exercise, since doing that lifts our spirits and keeps our body working well. Also keep in mind that when you first got your period, you would have shifts in your mood and people would say it was because you were going through adolescence. Back then, your changing hor-*

mones were the excuse or reason given to explain your behavior. Later, when you had regular periods, your mood shifts were attributed to your being premenstrual or having premenstrual syndrome (PMS). In menopause you will go through mood shifts again. When you get to be post-menopausal, you will be free of hormonal mood swings, and you may find that you are more clearheaded.

- *YOU EXPERIENCE TROUBLE FOCUSING, "FUZZY THINKING," OR FORGETFULNESS. While some women attribute such experiences to menopause, they probably are more a function of lack of sleep. The data indicate that menopause has little impact on memory or related functions. If you continue to have problems in this area, you need to discuss the issue with your health care provider to make sure that there is not another health issue needing attention.*

Q Will I feel better?
Of course you will. Just like you survived going through the changes of adolescence, you will get through menopause, since it is just at the other end of the hormonal continuum. And the good part is that once you are post-menopausal, you do not have to worry about birth control. Sexual intimacy and lovemaking can continue to be joyful.

Q What if someone I know is going through menopause?
Try to be patient with her, because her internal thermostat is going through some major adjustments. You can help by making healthy meals, supporting her fitness activities, and trying to create that sleep sanctuary for her.

You can also help her feel physically comfortable. You may want to wear a sweater, as she may want the room to be at a temperature that is too cool for you. Remember that there is a limit as to how many layers the person going through menopause can take off, whereas you can always add layers. You can also celebrate going sleeveless.

WHERE TO LEARN MORE

NATIONAL INSTITUTE ON AGING
www.nia.nih.gov/HealthInformation/Publications/menopause.htm
The NIA is part of the NIH, and it provides extensive information on menopause.

NATIONAL LIBRARY OF MEDICINE (NLM): MEDLINEPLUS
www.nlm.nih.gov/medlineplus/menopause.html
The NLM is the library resource for NIH, and it provides news, as well as information on therapy, clinical trials, research, and other resources related to menopause.

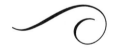

Menstruation

"It would be so much easier if I didn't have to think about periods."

LATINAS AND MENSTRUATION

- *Latinas menstruate earlier than non-Hispanic white girls do.*

- *Latinas are less likely to have a condition in which the ovary does not release a ripened egg each month (anovulation) than non-Hispanic white women do.*

Q *Que pasa?*
During their childbearing years, healthy women have menstrual cycles; when women are undernourished or stressed, they stop having menstrual cycles. Your menstruation, or period, is part of who you are. Fortunately, we do not live in a place or time when menstruation is seen as unclean or we are banished to a menstrual hut. Menstruation is part of being a woman. Menarche is your first period, and it is one of the later signs of puberty.

For most women in the United States, menstruation begins between the ages of eight and fifteen, with the average age of onset being twelve. As discussed earlier, the end of menstruation is menopause, when women no longer have periods and they cannot get pregnant. A clear understanding of menstruation helps us appreciate what happens with our ovaries, fallopian tubes, uterus, cervix, and vagina.

The story of menstruation begins in our ovaries. Our ovaries are more than the keeper of all the eggs that we will

MYTH: When you wear tight pants, other people can see your vagina.
FACT: The vagina is an internal organ.

MYTH: When you have your period, it is better not to exercise.
FACT: For some women, exercising during their period reduces their cramps.

ever have; they are also endocrine glands responsible for the hormonal dance that produces our menstrual cycle. The menstrual cycle, which is under the direction of the endocrine system, involves several steps:

Follicular phase: Estrogen is released by the ovaries, and this causes the thickening of the walls of the uterus.

Ovulation: When one of your ovaries releases an egg, it travels through the fallopian tubes and to the uterus. This process is called ovulation, and the luteinizing hormone (LH) that is released by your pituitary gland plays a key role in the process. This is when you are most likely to get pregnant—three days before ovulation or on the day of ovulation.

Luteal phase: Progesterone is released and prepares the walls of the uterus so that a fertilized egg can become attached.

Menstruation: This is when you actually bleed. If, after about two weeks (ten to sixteen days), a fertilized egg does not attach itself to the walls of the uterus, there is a sharp drop in progesterone and estrogen. The uterus sheds the lining that had accumulated to hold the fertilized egg. That is why sometimes some of your period will look a little bit more chunky than liquid. The lining passes through the cervix and into the vagina and either comes out through your vaginal opening or is absorbed by a tampon that is in your vagina.

PROBLEMS AND PREVENTION

Sometimes the problems women experience with their periods are more severe than the typical cramping or tired feeling. Here are the major problems that can occur:

Amenorrhea: This is the term used to describe the condition when women do not get their period. Specifically, it includes teens aged fifteen or older who have never had a period, as well as women who menstruate but who have gone ninety days without a period. Sometimes missing periods is due to extreme weight loss, eating disorders, excessive exercising, or stress. It also can signal the occurrence of hormonal issues such as polycystic ovarian syndrome (PCOS) or other problems.

Dysmenorrhea: This is when periods are very painful and include severe cramps. Generally, for younger women severe cramps are not a sign of disease but are due to the production of prostaglandin as part of the menstrual cycle. As women get older, the same symptoms may indicate uterine fibroids or endometriosis. Both of these conditions require the attention of your health care provider.

186

Abnormal uterine bleeding: The only way to know what is abnormal is to have a good idea of what your output is like when you are menstruating. You need to be familiar with your menstrual bleeding so that you can tell when it is different from what it normally looks like. Keeping a menstrual chart is a good habit. Record the amount of flow, the color, and the thickness. This will help you and your health care provider determine what may be happening and develop a treatment plan for you.

Toxic shock syndrome (TSS): The women who have died from this infection became ill because they had not changed their tampon for a long time and had introduced bacteria into their vagina. To avoid TSS, make sure to wash your hands before inserting a tampon. Also, follow these recommendations from the Food and Drug Administration (FDA):

- *Follow package directions for insertion.*

- *Choose the lowest absorbency that is appropriate for your flow.*

- *Change your tampon at least every four to eight hours.*

- *Consider alternating pads with tampons.*

- *Know the warning signs of TSS—sudden high fever over 102 degrees, muscle aches, diarrhea, vomiting, dizziness and/or fainting, sunburn-like rash, sore throat, bloodshot eyes.*

- *Do not use tampons between periods.*

HEALTH POINT

Tampons should be changed every four to eight hours to avoid getting toxic shock syndrome (TSS).

187

Q Can I get better?
Menstruation is not an illness or a disease. It is one of the functions of a healthy woman's body during part of her lifetime. Being a woman is about having hormones.

Q What if someone I know is having her period?
If she is having cramps, you can offer to get her a heated blanket or go for a walk together. Each of us gets through cramps in our own way. And of course there is always chocolate.

WHERE TO LEARN MORE

OFFICE ON WOMEN'S HEALTH
www.womenshealth.gov
This government website offers up-to-date information on menstruation and the menstrual cycle.

NATIONAL LIBRARY OF MEDICINE (NLM): MEDLINE PLUS
www.nlm.nih.gov/medlineplus/menstruation
The NLM is the library resource for the NIH and has up-to-date information for consumers.

NATIONAL INSTITUTE OF CHILD HEALTH AND HUMAN DEVELOPMENT (NICHD)
www.nichd.nih.gov
The NICHD is the primary NIH organization for research on menstruation.

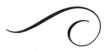

Pregnancy

"I know I'm pregnant, but I don't feel pregnant."

LATINAS AND PREGNANCY

- *Latinas are the women least likely to die from an illness related to or made worse by pregnancy or the care during pregnancy.*

- *Latinas have a higher rate of getting gestational diabetes than other women have.*

———

Q *Que pasa?*
One Latina told me how weird it was that in the past women wore maternity clothes to hide their growing belly. Now, women wear maternity clothes that accentuate their bodily changes. While today's woman wants to be in control, plan her pregnancy, and let others know of her baby's growth, unplanned pregnancies still occur sometimes. This means we have to live healthily in order to be prepared for the unplanned.

As discussed earlier, none of the methods for temporary birth control is 100 percent effective, except for abstinence from vaginal sex. Given that pregnancy is a possibility, the best way to be prepared is to make health and fitness part of your daily life now. Specifically, you have to not smoke *and* stay away from smoke, eat healthy foods, stay fit, do all you can to have a positive and happy attitude, and limit how much alcohol you drink. These are the same principles you would follow if you were pregnant, with the exception that you would not drink any alcohol during pregnancy.

When you are pregnant, whatever you take into your body—chemicals through your skin, smoke you breathe, alcohol you

> **MYTH:** You should start prenatal care when you do not feel well.
>
> **FACT:** Start prenatal care as soon as possible. While the ideal time to start thinking about your pregnancy is before you are pregnant, you should see your health care provider as soon as you think you are pregnant.
>
> ---
>
> **MYTH:** The first three months of pregnancy are not very important.
>
> **FACT:** The first three months are very important for the baby's healthy development.

drink, or food you eat—will affect your baby. For example, we know that smoking results in smaller babies because it cuts the flow of blood to the baby. We also know that what you feel will influence your baby's development.

So rather than focusing on a laundry list of what you should or should not do, just get into the mindset that you are carrying very precious cargo that needs to be cared for in special ways by you and those near you.

ABOUT FOLIC ACID

Folic acid is a manmade substance that has the same positive effects as folate, which is a vitamin naturally found in many foods. Some foods high in folate are beans, lentils, peas, juices, fruits, nuts, and dark green vegetables. When we do not get enough folate, we may feel tired or get headaches, and our skin may be lose its luster. All of these may be signs of anemia. Folate is so important that in May 2009 the U.S. Preventive Services Task Force recommended that all women planning or capable of pregnancy take a daily supplement containing 0.4 to 0.8 mg (400 to 800 micrograms) of folic acid. If you are thinking of getting pregnant or are pregnant, remember that folate will help your baby have a healthy spine and brain. Women in general need to consume 400 micrograms (mcg) of folic acid (in pill form) each day, and you should consume another 400 mcg per day through your diet.

Q *Do I have a problem? Now what?*
For most Latinas, pregnancy is a blessing, albeit a mixed blessing at times. Nevertheless, when you are planning to become pregnant or as soon as you think you are pregnant, you should visit your prenatal care provider. Although pregnancy lasts for about forty weeks, the sooner you schedule this visit the better it is for you and your baby.

During the first seven months (twenty-eight weeks) of your pregnancy you will see your prenatal care provider about once a month. You will go for more visits as you get closer to your due date. If your prenatal care provider has concerns about your health or your baby's health, you may have more frequent visits. Your weight will be monitored to make sure that you gain the right amount of weight and to make sure that all is going well with you and the baby.

During your first visit, your prenatal care provider will talk to you and confirm all the information about your health and your habits, conduct a physical exam and a series of tests (blood, urine, Pap, and tests for STDs), and calculate your due date. If you had gestational diabetes during previous pregnancies, have diabetes in your family, or have given birth to large babies, it is likely that your blood sugar will be tested during your first visit. For other women the test for diabetes is given during the visit that is between the twenty-fourth and twenty-eighth weeks of pregnancy.

If you are over thirty-five or the baby is at risk of having a genetic disorder, your prenatal care provider may suggest more tests. For example, during weeks ten to twelve, chorionic villus sampling (CVS) may be recommended. This test is done by inserting a needle through your belly or a catheter into your cervix to get cells from the placenta. In this test the cells drawn from the placenta are tested for Down's syndrome and other genetic illnesses. Another test that may be recommended is amniocentesis during weeks fourteen to eighteen. Both of these tests carry a small risk of miscarriage.

During weeks eighteen to twenty your health care provider will use ultrasound technology to produce a picture of the baby. By looking at this image, your prenatal care provider will be able to see how the baby is growing and give a better estimate of where you are in your pregnancy. Although the ultrasound is considered safe, repeating it is not recommended unless it is medically necessary. At about weeks eighteen to twenty-two the baby will move more, and you may even feel kicking.

There may be times after your twentieth week when you experience cramps and contractions in your uterus. These are called Braxton Hicks contractions, and they are mini labor contractions. They are short and mild, and they do not have a pattern. As the weeks go by, you may have some more of these, but they are different from labor. When you are in labor, the contractions are more frequent and more uncomfortable, and they follow a pattern. In any case, if you note any regular contractions or pain, you should contact your health care provider immediately.

In addition to your regular visits there are times when it is important to contact your prenatal care provider even though you do not have a scheduled visit. You should call your prenatal care provider if you have symptoms such as vaginal bleeding; swollen hands and feet; severe headaches that will not go away; blurred vision or the sense that someone has dimmed the lights; back, stomach, or pelvic pain that does not go away; a change in the number or types of movements the baby makes; painful or burning urination; or a major change

HEALTH POINT

Do not handle kitty litter during pregnancy, as microscopic pieces of cat feces can give you a parasite that can delay the development of the baby's brain and affect the eyes. That is why it is also good to use gloves when gardening.

in how you are feeling. Make sure to talk with a person in the prenatal care provider's office (instead of leaving a message on a machine) to determine whether you need to make an appointment. And if you cannot talk with someone there, then go to the emergency room for immediate attention.

Q What if someone I know is pregnant?
Your best role is to be supportive of the mother and the baby. Try to help her as she adjusts to her ever-changing body and her needs for comfort. Help her to eat healthily, stay away from smoke and alcohol, be as fit as she can, and enjoy her pregnancy. The best thing you can do for someone who is pregnant is to bring laughter into her life and remind her of how wonderful she looks.

WHERE TO LEARN MORE

NATIONAL HISPANIC PRENATAL HELPLINE • 1-800-504-7081
This exceptional bilingual service can direct you to a health care provider and send you free information to help you have a healthy baby. This is a program of the National Alliance for Hispanic Health. The service is available Monday through Friday from 9:00 to 6:00 p.m., Eastern Standard Time.

NATIONAL INSTITUTE FOR CHILD HEALTH
AND HUMAN DEVELOPMENT (NICHD)
   www.nichd.nih.gov
The NICHD, which is part of the NIH, supports and conducts research on topics related to the health of children, adults, families, and populations.

Sex, Sexuality, and Sexual Intimacy

"I can't talk about that."

LATINAS AND SEXUALITY

- *Latinas are the women least likely to have problems having an orgasm.*
- *Seventy percent of Latinas do not lack interest in sex.*

Q *Que pasa?*
It must be the puritanical roots of the United States, compounded by some misplaced taboos, but there are relatively few studies about sex (the mechanics), sexuality (how we feel about ourselves and nurture and express those feelings), or sexual intimacy (how we share ourselves with others). The few large national studies are almost two decades old and our views have changed dramatically since those studies. Television, movies, and the web are filled with sexual images and messages that range from subtle to screaming about sex. And while there is plenty of sexual content in what we are exposed to the views of sex being presented are as unreal and distorted as the Photoshop-tweaked images of silicone-inflated female breasts that are the standard. There is little media coverage that is truly informative and helpful. Making matters worse, many of us are reluctant to admit what we don't know and thus we perpetuate the myth that we already know what we need to know.

That we are confused about the proper place for sex in society and for expressing and sharing our sexuality should not be a surprise. Think about the mixed messages that society gives children. At the same time that we are rightfully appalled at all types of sexual abuse of children, some parents think it is cute to

MYTH:	Oral sex is not sex.
FACT:	Oral sex is sex, and it may also be part of sexual intimacy. While you may not get pregnant, you can get STDs.
MYTH:	Sexuality is about having lots of partners.
FACT:	Sexuality is about how you feel about yourself.

buy eight- and nine-year-old girls T-shirts and clothing bearing sexually provocative words. Other parents may be uncertain, confused, or even uncomfortable about the physical and other changes their daughters are experiencing during puberty. Puberty for girls means that their bodies are getting ready for childbirth. While their bodies are driving them to believe that they are no longer children, the fluctuations in their hormones are taking their emotions to all sorts of highs and lows. To complicate matters, girls are reaching puberty at a younger age due to a variety of factors, which may even include environmental pollutants that are affecting how our children mature physically. And for young Latinas, all of these issues are compounded by the challenge of blending the values of their Hispanic and non-Hispanic worlds. The consequences of this are huge. We know that girls born outside of the U.S. mainland are likely to engage in sexual activity later than girls born in the United States are.

CAUSES AND PREVENTION

If it was hard growing up when girls were expected to assume fairly limited roles, it is even harder now when girls and women are given the wrong messages about how to express themselves sexually. The "popular girls" in most of the media images are the ones who seem to use sex as social currency, and this becomes even more pronounced as those girls get older and become the hottest new images of what is a sexy woman.

195

No matter the age, it is breast and butt size, not brainpower, being portrayed as mattering for girls and women. This hype continues even though women know that many of the media images have been developed by men with little or no interest in portraying what is real, healthy, or good for women.

It is essential to help all women have healthy views about sex and positive self-images. That is why we have to talk about sex—the broad topic that includes everything from biology to mechanics. At the same time the most important role for all women—mothers, *tías* (aunts), *abuelas* (grandmothers), and so on—is to model healthy sexuality and sexual intimacy throughout all ages.

Your sexuality has to do with how much you enjoy your own skin, scent, and texture; your sexual orientation; and your feelings about men and women. It is reflected in everything you do. When you are conflicted, confused, or disturbed about your own sexuality, these feelings are also reflected in what you do. Healthy sexuality is about doing what feels good for you and what feels nourishing. It includes everything from wearing clothes where the fabric feels good on your skin to enjoying the feeling of warm bathwater.

Sexual intimacy is about sharing the good feelings about your body, mind, and spirit with someone else. It is so much more than the tension-reduction type of sexual release you can get from masturbating or from having sex with someone. The intimacy factor is what changes the nature of arousal and sexual communication. Intimacy is a shared experience. It is about the strength and the caring that you and your partner share with each other. There is no one definition that will be applicable to every person, since the nuances are what make intimate experiences unique. There are some steps we can take to have healthy attitudes about these important areas.

HEALTH POINT

Sexual intimacy should not involve pain or discomfort.

First, we have to accept the idea that sex, sexuality, and sexual intimacy are part of our human uniqueness. Whether we consider sex a gift from God or part of the randomness of life is not the issue. The goal is to see sex as part of the positive aspect of who we are.

Second, we have to embrace our own sexuality. That does not mean we should go and "strut our stuff." It means that we recognize who we are as sexual beings. Parents should be particularly aware that children who are raised in families that are not supportive of their sexuality and sexual orientation are more likely to have problems. Moreover, these children grow up to be adults who are conflicted until their own issues are resolved. Finally, we have to appreciate that sexual intimacy should be joyful and we deserve that it should be a part of our life.

Q Do I have a problem?
Healthy relationships in the past are the best predictors of healthy relationships in the future, but some women have not been fortunate in that way. Consequently, for some women, they do not have sexual intimacy, but rather they have sex that is devoid of intimacy; it is merely something they do. And while a woman may be happy with such an approach, assuming that she has a partner whom she enjoys and who actively desires her, it may be a signal that other issues need to be sorted out.

Women who have had sexual trauma in their lives may have problems with their own feelings about sex, sexuality, and sexual intimacy. For these women the first protective barrier they set up is either to deny that the trauma ever happened or to sever the relationship between feelings and sex. Sexuality becomes more than social currency; for some it becomes real currency as well. It is not surprising that many women who are in the sex industry were sexually abused as children.

This is a very difficult subject, since the very nature of the trauma creates emotional conflict and distorts the woman's view of her body and relationship to her own pleasure. Some women who have been sexually abused are able to get beyond the damage that was done to them by recognizing, most importantly, that the abuse was not their fault and that the perpetrator was disturbed. A woman's recognition of not having been at fault is critical, because most abusers are skilled at making the person who was abused believe that what happened was her fault. Often, women who have been sexually abused need professional help to address the disturbances in their lives created by the abuse.

Q Will it get better?
Yes. If the problem has to do with your own sexual expression and pleasure, there is much you can do, assuming that you have a willing partner. Sex therapy for couples can be very effective. Sometimes, however, the problem to be resolved is out of your control. This is especially true when your partner is the one who has unresolved issues and does not want to seek help.

Q What if someone I know has a problem
related to sexuality?
It depends on what her problem is. Latinas talking to each other are a great source of support. But sometimes we seem to avoid the details that define our discomfort because we do not want to show our own ignorance or lack of experience. We need to listen with our *corazón* (heart) as we encourage our *amiga* to seek professional help to accept her sexuality and the goal of sexual intimacy.

WHERE TO LEARN MORE

NATIONAL INSTITUTE ON AGING (NIA)
www.niapublications.org/agepages/sexuality.asp
The NIA, which is part of the NIH, has much information on sexuality
in later life.

NEMOURS FOUNDATION: KIDS HEALTH FOR PARENTS
kidshealth.org/parent/growth/sexual_health/development.html
This not-for-profit foundation has information for parents on the
early sexual development of children.

PARENTS, FAMILIES, AND FRIENDS OF LESBIANS AND GAYS
community.pflag.org/Page.aspx?pid=594
This national nonprofit organization is a vast grassroots network
with more than 200,000 members and more than 500 affiliates in
the United States.

NATIONAL SEXUAL ASSAULT HOTLINE
www.rainn.org/get-help/national-sexual-assault-hotline
Call 1-800-656-HOPE to speak to a counselor. The call is anonymous
and confidential.

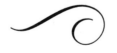

Sexually Transmitted Diseases (STDs) or Sexually Transmitted Infections (STIs)

"I don't have any symptoms, so I know I'm okay."

LATINAS AND STDs

- *In 2007, the chlamydia rate among Latinas was three times higher than the rate among whites.*

- *In 2007, the gonorrhea rate among Latinas was higher than the rate among whites.*

Q *Que pasa?*
Latinas have low rates of condom use and high rates of STDs. We need to start protecting ourselves and each other because STDs are serious. The various ones are caused by either bacteria, viruses, or parasites. Many times the person who gets an STD has no symptoms. For example, almost nine out of ten people who have genital herpes do not know they have it. The only way to know if you have been exposed is to get tested.

Some STDs may be cured with antibiotics, and others can only be treated. In all cases consistent and correct use of condoms provides some protection from STDs. In most cases STDs that are untreated can create problems ranging from pelvic inflammatory disease to infertility to cancer. You should get tested for STDs if either you or your partner have been or are sexually active with others.

> **MYTH:** You can look at people and know whether they have an STD.
> **FACT:** You cannot tell by looking at people whether they have an STD.
>
> ---
>
> **MYTH:** If I use a condom, I am protected from STDs.
> **FACT:** Condoms offer substantial but not 100 percent protection.

CAUSES AND PREVENTION

What follows are the most common STDs (listed in alphabetical order) and the key facts about them. HIV/AIDS is also considered an STD and is discussed in its own section.

CHLAMYDIA

CAUSE: Chlamydia is caused by bacteria that act like a virus because they cannot reproduce without a host.

SYMPTOMS: There are usually none. Some women may have an unusual discharge from the vagina or burning during urination. If you have had anal sex, you may have pain, bleeding, or a discharge from your rectum.

PREVENTION: Consistent and correct use of latex condoms greatly reduces the risk of catching or spreading chlamydia.

WHO GETS IT: Women and men can get this STD, plus babies born to infected mothers can get eye infections and pneumonia.

IMPACTS: Chlamydia affects the genital areas, the mouth, or the anus.

TESTING: Your health care provider will take a swab sample from your cervix or a urine sample (which is much less accurate for women than it is for men) and send it to a lab for analysis. Sometimes a urine test will also be done to see if bacteria are present. You should be tested once a year if you are twenty-five or younger and are having sex, older than twenty-five and with more than one sexual partner or with any new sexual partners, or if you are pregnant.

TREATMENT: Chlamydia is cured with antibiotics. If untreated, it leads to serious health problems, including infertility.

GONORRHEA

CAUSE: Bacteria cause gonorrhea.

SYMPTOMS: There are not always symptoms. In women it can cause bleeding between periods, pain when urinating, and increased discharge from the vagina.

PREVENTION: Consistent and correct use of latex condoms greatly reduces the risk of catching or spreading this STD.

WHO GETS IT: Women, men, and babies born to infected mothers can get it.

IMPACTS: The genital areas, the mouth, the throat, or the anus can be affected.

TESTING: A simple lab test is used.

TREATMENT: Most of the time gonorrhea can be cured with antibiotics, but there are new strains that cannot be cured with existing antibiotics. If untreated, it can lead to pelvic inflammatory disease, which causes problems with pregnancy and infertility. Among people with gonorrhea, 1 percent develop a type of arthritis.

HERPES SIMPLEX VIRUS TYPE 2 (HSV-2);

also called HSV or genital herpes

CAUSE: HSV-2 is caused by a virus.

SYMPTOMS: There are not always symptoms. Some people may get sores near the area where the virus has entered the body. The sores blister, become itchy and painful, and then heal.

PREVENTION: Consistent and correct use of latex condoms can reduce your risk of catching or spreading HSV-2, but it does not cover all the areas. Abstain if your partner has an outbreak of herpes.

HEALTH POINT

The herpes simplex virus type 1 (HSV-1) that causes cold sores around your mouth can be transmitted to the genital area through oral sex.

Who gets it: Women and men can get HSV-2. Also, babies whose mothers have HSV-2 can get it during childbirth.

Impact: The genitals, the buttocks, or the anal area can be affected. You may get several outbreaks a year, though they occur less often over time. Sometimes there will be no visible signs, but the virus will be on your skin's surface and will be highly contagious.

Testing: A swab is taken of a fresh sore, and the cells are analyzed in either of two ways. They may be put in a special container (cell culture cup) and allowed to multiply, so that they can be examined under a microscope, or a solution may be added to the sample on the swab and examined under a microscope.

Treatment: There is no cure for HSV-2. Antiviral medicines can help lessen the symptoms and decrease outbreaks. If untreated, a person's symptoms may worsen, but they usually resolve on their own within ten to fourteen days.

HUMAN PAPILLOMAVIRUS (HPV)

Cause: The virus causing HPV has more than 100 strains.

Symptoms: HPV usually involves no symptoms, but some people develop genital warts.

Prevention: Consistent and correct use of latex condoms can reduce the risk of catching or spreading HPV. A vaccine is available to prevent (but not treat) the most common forms of HPV.

Who gets it: Women and men can get HPV.

Impact: Low-risk HPV can cause genital warts. High-risk HPV can lead to cancer.

Testing: Pap smears can detect HPV-related changes in the cervix that might lead to cancer. New tests for HPV were approved in 2009.

Treatment: A health care provider can treat or remove HPV-related warts. If HPV is untreated, the body sometimes will clear the infection; however, untreated HPV can lead to cancer of the cervix, vulva, vagina, and anus.

SYPHILIS

CAUSE: Bacteria cause syphilis.

SYMPTOMS: There are not always symptoms. The primary stage of syphilis usually causes a single, small, painless blister or sore (chancre) that disappears on its own. In the secondary stage, a rash and sores appear, especially on the palms of the hands and soles of the feet. Many people do not notice the symptoms for years.

PREVENTION: Avoid contact with an infected sore. Condoms cover only part of the area where there may be contact.

WHO GETS IT: Women and men can get syphilis, as can babies born to infected mothers. Mothers with undetected syphilis are at increased risk of losing their baby during pregnancy, or shortly after birth.

IMPACTS: The genital area, the lips, the mouth, or the anus can be affected.

TESTING: Syphilis is detected through a blood test or an examination of bacteria from infected sores.

TREATMENT: In the primary and secondary stages syphilis can be treated with antibiotics. If untreated, it will advance to the tertiary (late) stage, meaning it will spread throughout your body and damage your major organs, causing paralysis, dementia, blindness, and death.

TRICHOMONIASIS

CAUSE: A parasite causes trichomoniasis.

SYMPTOMS: A green or yellow discharge from the vagina, an unpleasant smell from the vagina, itching in or near the vagina, and discomfort with urination may occur.

PREVENTION: Consistent and correct use of latex condoms reduces the risk of catching or spreading trichomoniasis.

WHO GETS IT: Both women and men can get this STD.

IMPACTS: The genital area.

TESTING: A sample of the discharge is put on a slide and examined.

TREATMENT: To treat trichomoniasis, you and your partner should be treated with antibiotics. If trichomoniasis is not treated, the symptoms will continue.

Q *What if someone I know has an STD?*
You should be examined by your health care provider as you may need treatment. If this is someone with whom you have had sexual contact then the two of you should discuss the steps needed to ensure that you both will be examined and treated by a health care provider. If you feel you cannot talk to the person, then you need to ask yourself whether it makes sense to engage in sexual activity with someone with whom you cannot have a serious conversation.

WHERE TO LEARN MORE

NATIONAL LIBRARY OF MEDICINE (NLM): MEDLINE PLUS
www.nlm.nih.gov/medlineplus/sexuallytransmitteddiseases.html
The NLM is the library resource of the NIH, and it offers links to news and articles on sexually transmitted diseases, as well as news about such things as Internet-advertised drugs that falsely claim to prevent treat STDs.

CDC—SEXUALLY TRANSMITTED DISEASES
www.cdc.gov/std
The CDC information includes statistics about and treatment guidelines for sexually transmitted diseases (STDs), along with referrals to STD clinics.

AMERICAN SOCIAL HEALTH ASSOCIATION
www.ashastd.org/learn/learn
This not-for-profit organization is dedicated to informing the public about STDs.

Glossary of Frequently Used Words

Sometimes we may feel fairly certain about the meaning of words that we come across when we read health news or have discussions with our health care provider, only to find out later that the meaning is very different from what we thought. The following section contains my selection of the most commonly used health-related words for which you need to know the accurate meaning.

CARDIOVASCULAR DISEASE: This includes high blood pressure, high cholesterol, and heart disease. What these conditions have in common is that they cause your arteries to get narrow (constrict), which leads to the heart getting less blood.

CHOLESTEROL: Cholesterol is essential in helping your body properly absorb fat, as well as vitamins A, D, E, and K. But too much cholesterol is not good, since it increases your risk of having a heart attack. Your cholesterol level is given as a total number that indicates your level of low density lipoprotein (LDL) and high density lipoprotein (HDL). LDL is believed to be the main source of cholesterol buildup and blockage in the arteries, so you want to keep the amount of it low. HDL helps keep cholesterol from building up in the arteries, so you want to keep the level of it high.

CLINICAL TRIAL: This is a study you may choose to participate in so that researchers can find out more about the effectiveness of a treatment or intervention. There are different kinds of clinical trials, but all of them require your informed consent. Each clinical trial has specific guidelines about what criteria someone must meet to be included (e.g., a certain age range), as well as what characteristics would exclude someone from a clinical trial (e.g., having already had certain treatments for a condition). For in-depth information, look at *clinicaltrials.gov*, and for information on cancer-related clinical trials call 1-800-4-Cancer.

Endocrine system: This is a system of glands located throughout your body, and it includes the hypothalamus, pituitary gland, thyroid, parathyroid glands, adrenal glands, pineal body, ovaries, testes, and pancreas. Each of these glands makes and releases (secretes) specific hormones. Fat cells are also part of the endocrine system, as there are hormones that have been found to originate there. The endocrine system plays a key role in diabetes.

HDL: See cholesterol.

Hormones: Hormones are the body's chemical messengers. They work slowly and affect every part of the body. They are produced and regulated by the endocrine system.

Hysterectomy: This is the most common surgery in the United States (excluding cesarean section delivery). Depending on the reason for the surgery, it may involve removal of the ovaries, fallopian tubes, uterus (all or parts), cervix, upper part of the vagina, and supporting tissue. Research has shown that there are health benefits to leaving your ovaries even if other parts are removed. A hysterectomy may be recommended as one of the ways to treat fibroids, endometriosis, cancer, and other conditions. Recovery varies by the age and fitness of the woman, as well as by whether the surgery involves cutting through your abdominal area (six to eight weeks for recovery), going through your vagina (four to six weeks), or making a very small cut and using a device called a laparoscope (three to six weeks).

Full recovery takes time, so make sure to adjust your planned activities accordingly. Once your uterus is removed, you will not be able to get pregnant. If your ovaries are removed, you will begin menopause.

INCIDENCE: This refers to the number of new cases occurring over a certain period of time, usually a year. The incidence rate gives you an idea of the risk of getting a condition over the specified period of time. For some conditions, such as arthritis, you cannot know the incidence, since the condition develops over time.

LDL: See cholesterol.

METABOLIC SYNDROME: This is a relatively new diagnosis for a cluster of conditions that increase your risk for diabetes and heart disease. These conditions include high blood pressure, blood sugar levels, and triglycerides; low levels of HDL; and too much fat in the belly area.

MORBIDITY: This term refers to sickness, and it is used to give information about people who have a condition or are sick. Morbidity rate refers to the proportion or percentage of people who are sick. The more morbidity, the sicker you are; the less the morbidity, the healthier you are.

MORTALITY: This term refers to death or having died. Mortality rate refers to the proportion or percentage of people who have died or are dying from a condition. An increase in mortality means more people are dying; a decrease means fewer people are dying.

OSTEOPOROSIS: This is when your bones get weak and then become more likely to break. More than half of women over age fifty have osteoporosis. To reduce the likelihood of getting osteoporosis, women need to take calcium supplements and vitamin D (from direct exposure to sunlight and from foods such as fortified milk, egg yolks, saltwater fish, and liver) and to do weight-bearing exercises (weight training, walking, climbing stairs, dancing). Remember that your bones are alive, and exercise helps them and your muscles get stronger.

OXYTOCIN: Sometimes called the love hormone, this is a hormone in the brain that has a role with respect to emotional bonds, sex, childbirth, and breastfeeding.

POSITIVE RESULTS: This means that you do have whatever you have been tested for. It may be good news (e.g., you want to be pregnant and you tested positive) or bad news (e.g., you do not want to be pregnant and you tested positive).

PREVALENCE: This refers to how many people actually have a condition. Sometimes prevalence is expressed as a percentage or as a proportion of the population.

RISK: This means the likelihood that something will happen. The risk that any of us will die at some point is 100 percent. The risk that any of us will never have a single infection of any kind is 0 percent. To know what a risk means to you personally, you need to know what the original level of risk is and what the value of taking that risk is.

Very often in health-related discussions you hear that doing something in particular will double your risk of getting a specific condition. Let's say your original risk was 1 percent, or 1 out of 100. If you doubled the risk, then your risk would be 2 percent, or 2 out of 100. If the original risk was 25 percent, then doubling the risk means you would have a 50 percent chance of getting the condition. Your decision about whether to take a particular risk depends on what you are considering.

For example, if you had a terminal illness and there was an experimental treatment that extended life for 2 percent (2 out of 100) of the people treated, you might decide to take the risk and try it. If it extended life for only .1 percent (1 out of 1,000 people), you might decide not to try it.

SURVIVAL RATE: This represents the number of people who are alive after a fixed period of time. For most cancers, the term survival rate refers to the number of people who are alive five years after diagnosis. For other diseases, the number of years may vary. This term does not refer to the quality of life for people who have survived any specific disease.

TRIGGER: This is something that sets off another reaction. For example, air pollutants can trigger asthma and other respiratory problems.

TRIGLYCERIDES: This is a form of fat that is produced by the body and that can come from the food we eat.

RECORD KEEPING AND RESOURCES

Part Three

WHILE HAVING INFORMATION IS IMPORTANT, THERE ARE some key tools that can help you be in control of your health. The tools and guidelines in this part of the book will help you be accurate, informed, and organized for all the health decisions you must make for yourself and your family. "Record Keeping and Resources" provides the following:

"About My Health" is, in effect, a five-part tool you can use to track your own health. It contains the following parts:

- *My Health Overview*
- *Visits to My Health Care Provider*
- *How I Feel*
- *It's My Period*
- *My Medicines, Vitamins, Supplements, Teas, and Other Things I Take*

All of these are forms you can use regularly to note important things about your health. For additional copies of all these forms, you can download them from http://www.hispanichealth.org/latinaguide/.

Making My Choices Now and Making Them Known is a set of guidelines about discussing the kind of care you want at all stages of your life and helping identify who can make the decisions on your behalf if you cannot do so yourself.

You Need to Ask to Know contains the questions you may want to discuss with your health care provider.

More Resources is a list of other health-related information you may find especially helpful.

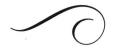

About My Health: Five Essential Tools

MEMORY IS WONDERFUL, BUT IT IS NOT THE BEST SOURCE OF accurate information, especially regarding your health and wellness. And while health care providers are increasingly using electronic health records, you also need to keep your own up-to-date records as a reference and a backup. "About My Health" is a set of five tools to help you stay informed about your health and track how you are feeling:

1. **MY HEALTH OVERVIEW** contains a summary sheet of basic information about your health and test results: blood pressure, weight, HDL, LDL, total cholesterol, triglycerides, and results from urine tests; and space to add information about other important points such as your iron levels or vaccinations you have had. The chart provides a quick overview of how you are doing.

2. **VISITS TO MY HEALTH CARE PROVIDER** is the summary of your visits, so that you can keep track of which health care providers you saw and when, what they said to you, and what medicines they prescribed.

3. **HOW I FEEL** provides a way for you to keep track of how your body feels and how your moods change. If you fill it in regularly, and especially when you are not feeling well, you will be able to provide your health care provider with timely and valuable information that can help in your diagnosis and in the development of a treatment plan for you. You can also use this part to see what factors change how your body feels or what your overall mood is. After a while you may notice that there are certain patterns to how your body and mind work, and you may find that certain activities or people are associated with your not feeling okay. It is good to be able to identify what is helpful and what is damaging in our lives.

To make it easier for you to describe your sense about your overall mood and how well your body feels, use this set of symbols:

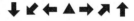

They range from extremely negative ↓ (down arrow) to extremely positive ↑ (up arrow). The meaning of each symbol is as follows:

↓ = extremely negative (bad)

↙ = moderately negative (very cranky)

← = slightly negative (cranky)

▲ = neutral (okay)

→ = slightly positive (good)

↗ = moderately positive (very good)

↑ = extremely positive (excellent)

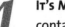 **IT'S MY PERIOD** contains a chart on which you can keep information about your menstrual flow and your moods.

5. **MEDICINES, VITAMINS, SUPPLEMENTS, TEAS, AND OTHER THINGS I TAKE** provides you a way to keep track of your prescription medicines, plus all the other things you take each day to influence your health.

The "About My Health" set of tools is to help you be organized. Be as honest as you can, and you will find it helpful in taking control of your health. When you have to take care of someone else, you can also use the "About My Health" resources to help keep track of what that person is experiencing.

My Health Overview

ABOUT ME _____

MY BLOOD TYPE _____   ALLERGIES _____

DATE	BLOOD PRESSURE	WEIGHT	HDL	LDL	TOTAL CHOLESTEROL	TRIGLYCERIDES	URINE	OTHER
	/							
	/							
	/							
	/							
	/							
	/							
	/							
	/							
	/							
	/							
	/							
	/							
	/							
	/							
	/							
	/							
	/							

ᴠɪꜱɪᴛꜱ Tᴏ Mʏ Hᴇᴀʟᴛʜ Cᴀʀᴇ Pʀᴏᴠɪᴅᴇʀ

Dᴀᴛᴇ _____   Wʜʏ I Wᴇɴᴛ _____

Wʜᴏᴍ I Sᴀᴡ _____

Sᴘᴇᴄɪᴀʟ Tᴇꜱᴛꜱ? _____

Dɪᴀɢɴᴏꜱɪꜱ? _____

Rᴇꜰᴇʀʀᴇᴅ Eʟꜱᴇᴡʜᴇʀᴇ? _____

Mᴇᴅɪᴄɪɴᴇꜱ Pʀᴇꜱᴄʀɪʙᴇᴅ _____

Wʜᴀᴛ Eʟꜱᴇ Dɪᴅ Tʜᴇ Hᴇᴀʟᴛʜ Cᴀʀᴇ Pʀᴏᴠɪᴅᴇʀ Dᴏ / Sᴀʏ? _____
_____
_____
_____

Dᴀᴛᴇ _____   Wʜʏ I Wᴇɴᴛ _____

Wʜᴏᴍ I Sᴀᴡ _____

Sᴘᴇᴄɪᴀʟ Tᴇꜱᴛꜱ? _____

Dɪᴀɢɴᴏꜱɪꜱ? _____

Rᴇꜰᴇʀʀᴇᴅ Eʟꜱᴇᴡʜᴇʀᴇ? _____

Mᴇᴅɪᴄɪɴᴇꜱ Pʀᴇꜱᴄʀɪʙᴇᴅ _____

Wʜᴀᴛ Eʟꜱᴇ Dɪᴅ Tʜᴇ Hᴇᴀʟᴛʜ Cᴀʀᴇ Pʀᴏᴠɪᴅᴇʀ Dᴏ / Sᴀʏ? _____
_____
_____
_____

⟋◯ How I Feel

DATE _____   MOOD: ↓ ↙ ← ▲ → ↗ ↑   BODY: ↓ ↙ ← ▲ → ↗ ↑

TEMPERATURE _____ AT _____ AM/PM

MY SYMPTOMS _____
_____
_____
_____
_____

OTHER CONCERNS _____
_____
_____
_____
_____
_____
_____

DATE _____   MOOD ↓ ↙ ← ▲ → ↗ ↑   BODY ↓ ↙ ← ▲ → ↗ ↑

TEMPERATURE _____ AT _____ AM/PM

MY SYMPTOMS _____
_____
_____
_____
_____

OTHER CONCERNS: _____
_____
_____
_____
_____
_____

⌒ IT'S MY PERIOD: FLOW AND MOOD

YEAR _____   FOR EACH DAY DESCRIBE YOUR FLOW USING THE FOLLOWING KEY:

MENSTRUAL FLOW: **S** = Spotting, **L** = Light, **M** = Medium, **H** = Heavy, **CH** = Chunky

MOOD: **B** = Bad, **CC** = Very Cranky, **C** = Cranky, **O** = Okay, **G** = Good, **GG** = Very Good, **E** = Excellent

JAN	FEB	MAR	APRIL	MAY	JUNE	JULY	AUG	SEPT	OCT	NOV	DEC
1	1	1	1	1	1	1	1	1	1	1	1
2	2	2	2	2	2	2	2	2	2	2	2
3	3	3	3	3	3	3	3	3	3	3	3
4	4	4	4	4	4	4	4	4	4	4	4
5	5	5	5	5	5	5	5	5	5	5	5
6	6	6	6	6	6	6	6	6	6	6	6
7	7	7	7	7	7	7	7	7	7	7	7
8	8	8	8	8	8	8	8	8	8	8	8
9	9	9	9	9	9	9	9	9	9	9	9
10	10	10	10	10	10	10	10	10	10	10	10
11	11	11	11	11	11	11	11	11	11	11	11
12	12	12	12	12	12	12	12	12	12	12	12
13	13	13	13	13	13	13	13	13	13	13	13
14	14	14	14	14	14	14	14	14	14	14	14
15	15	15	15	15	15	15	15	15	15	15	15
16	16	16	16	16	16	16	16	16	16	16	16
17	17	17	17	17	17	17	17	17	17	17	17
18	18	18	18	18	18	18	18	18	18	18	18
19	19	19	19	19	19	19	19	19	19	19	19
20	20	20	20	20	20	20	20	20	20	20	20
21	21	21	21	21	21	21	21	21	21	21	21
22	22	22	22	22	22	22	22	22	22	22	22
23	23	23	23	23	23	23	23	23	23	23	23
24	24	24	24	24	24	24	24	24	24	24	24
25	25	25	25	25	25	25	25	25	25	25	25
26	26	26	26	26	26	26	26	26	26	26	26
27	27	27	27	27	27	27	27	27	27	27	27
28	28	28	28	28	28	28	28	28	28	28	28
29	29	29	29	29	29	29	29	29	29	29	29
30		30	30	30	30	30	30	30	30	30	30
31		31		31		31	31		31		31

⌒◯ It's My Period: Flow and Mood

YEAR _____   FOR EACH DAY DESCRIBE YOUR FLOW USING THE FOLLOWING KEY:

MENSTRUAL FLOW: **S** = Spotting, **L** = Light, **M** = Medium, **H** = Heavy, **CH** = Chunky

MOOD: **B** = Bad, **CC** = Very Cranky, **C** = Cranky, **O** = Okay, **G** = Good, **GG** = Very Good, **E** = Excellent

JAN	FEB	MAR	APRIL	MAY	JUNE	JULY	AUG	SEPT	OCT	NOV	DEC
1	1	1	1	1	1	1	1	1	1	1	1
2	2	2	2	2	2	2	2	2	2	2	2
3	3	3	3	3	3	3	3	3	3	3	3
4	4	4	4	4	4	4	4	4	4	4	4
5	5	5	5	5	5	5	5	5	5	5	5
6	6	6	6	6	6	6	6	6	6	6	6
7	7	7	7	7	7	7	7	7	7	7	7
8	8	8	8	8	8	8	8	8	8	8	8
9	9	9	9	9	9	9	9	9	9	9	9
10	10	10	10	10	10	10	10	10	10	10	10
11	11	11	11	11	11	11	11	11	11	11	11
12	12	12	12	12	12	12	12	12	12	12	12
13	13	13	13	13	13	13	13	13	13	13	13
14	14	14	14	14	14	14	14	14	14	14	14
15	15	15	15	15	15	15	15	15	15	15	15
16	16	16	16	16	16	16	16	16	16	16	16
17	17	17	17	17	17	17	17	17	17	17	17
18	18	18	18	18	18	18	18	18	18	18	18
19	19	19	19	19	19	19	19	19	19	19	19
20	20	20	20	20	20	20	20	20	20	20	20
21	21	21	21	21	21	21	21	21	21	21	21
22	22	22	22	22	22	22	22	22	22	22	22
23	23	23	23	23	23	23	23	23	23	23	23
24	24	24	24	24	24	24	24	24	24	24	24
25	25	25	25	25	25	25	25	25	25	25	25
26	26	26	26	26	26	26	26	26	26	26	26
27	27	27	27	27	27	27	27	27	27	27	27
28	28	28	28	28	28	28	28	28	28	28	28
29	29	29	29	29	29	29	29	29	29	29	29
30		30	30	30	30	30	30	30	30	30	30
31		31		31		31	31		31		31

∽ My Medicines, Supplements, Teas, and Other Things I Take

NAME _____ COST _____

PURPOSE _____

SIZE / AMOUNT _____ COLOR _____ SHAPE _____

DATE PRESCRIBED_____ BY _____

HOW MUCH DO I TAKE? _____ WHEN? _____

THINGS TO AVOID _____

SIDE EFFECTS / OTHER COMMENTS _____

_____

_____

_____

_____

NAME _____ COST _____

PURPOSE _____

SIZE / AMOUNT _____ COLOR _____ SHAPE _____

DATE PRESCRIBED_____ BY _____

HOW MUCH DO I TAKE? _____ WHEN? _____

THINGS TO AVOID _____

SIDE EFFECTS / OTHER COMMENTS _____

_____

_____

_____

_____

Making My Choices Now and Making Them Known

TOO OFTEN WE LATINAS AVOID ANY DISCUSSION OF ADVANCE directives, or what we would or would not like done if we were so ill or impaired that we could not make our own decisions. Some of us fear that preparing advance directives will make something bad happen to us, and others of us are just uncomfortable with the topic. Yet it is important that we take control of our own health-related decision making while we are healthy and able to think clearly.

This is particularly important in the unlikely event that we are injured or incapacitated and unable to communicate what we want. That is why it is important to make sure your health care provider has in writing who can make these choices for you and what you want and do not want with respect to your own care.

A key step in making your preferences known is deciding whom you would trust to make critical health decisions on your behalf. If that person agrees to fulfill this role, she or he would become your designated health care agent or health care proxy, once you have indicated this choice in writing. Obviously, this is a very important decision. States have different laws about what you must do to make this designation. In most states your health care provider is legally prohibited from serving in this capacity.

While you may be very close to some family members or friends, you have to ask yourself the following questions about the person you are thinking of to fulfill this role:

1. Will she or he be willing to accept this role?
2. Is this person capable of making the commitment to this responsibility?
3. Will this person be physically available to meet the demands?
4. Does this person have the emotional strength to make the decisions that may be required?
5. Does this person know how to listen to you and know what you want?
6. Does this person have the ability to understand what health care providers are saying about your condition?
7. Will this person be able to talk to the other people who are close to you?
8. Is this person able to ask questions of the health care providers?
9. Does this person have any personal beliefs that would prevent her or him from meeting your requests?
10. Is this someone with whom you regularly communicate and someone who would know your wishes and desires?

Truthful answers to these questions may reveal that perhaps your spouse, relative, or your *comadre* may not be the best person to fulfill this role.

The conversation you have with the person you would like to designate should focus on conditions under which you would accept specific life-sustaining procedures and treatments, as well as your thoughts on end-of-life care. You may want your health care provider to discuss these procedures or treatments with you. Too often what we think these treatments involve is the relatively neat Hollywood portrayal of some of these procedures.

The National Hospice and Palliative Care Organization (NHPCO) has a program called Caring Connections with a website www.caringinfo.org. From the website you can download the advance directives that are legal in your state. You can do all of this without an attorney. You can also call the Caring Connections help line at 1-800-658-8898 or send an e-mail to them at caringinfo@nhpco.org.

Another way you can proceed is to use the Five Wishes set of forms, which were developed by Jim Towey, a wonderful, devout man who worked with Mother Teresa for twelve years. These forms (which are together in a booklet) are written in an easy-to-understand format to address a person's medical, personal, emotional, and spiritual needs. The Five Wishes forms meet the technical requirements of the respective laws of the following states. In some of these states there may be additional requirements, but those are included on the Five Wishes forms.

Alaska	Louisiana	North Dakota
Arizona	Maine	Oklahoma
Arkansas	Maryland	Pennsylvania
California	Massachusetts	Rhode Island
Colorado	Michigan	South Carolina
Connecticut	Minnesota	South Dakota
Delaware	Mississippi	Tennessee
District of Columbia	Missouri	Vermont
Florida	Montana	Virginia
Georgia	Nebraska	Washington
Hawaii	New Jersey	West Virginia
Idaho	New Mexico	Wisconsin
Illinois	New York	Wyoming
Iowa	North Carolina	

If your state does not accept the Five Wishes forms, then you may want to use them as a means of beginning a discussion. Your health care provider or local hospital may have some other form that meets the requirements of your state.

The Five Wishes forms, which are meant to be used by anyone eighteen or older, specifically address the following areas:

1. Selection of your health care agent (the person who will make decisions for you.) This cannot be your health care provider; an employee or spouse of an employee of your health care provider; or someone who serves as the health care agent role for ten or more people, unless that person is your spouse or close relative. The Five Wishes forms specify what the health care provider can and cannot decide, as well as what steps to take if you want to change your health care agent.
2. Statements of the kinds of treatment you will and will not want.
3. Statements of what you want done to make you feel comfortable.
4. Statements of how you want to be treated.
5. Statements for your loved ones.

You can get more information by calling toll-free at 1-888-5WISHES (1-888-594-7437) or by writing to Aging with Dignity, PO Box 1661, Tallahassee, FL 32302-1661. Cinco Deseos, the Spanish version of Five Wishes, is also available.

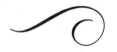

Knowing What I Need to Ask

Whenever you have an appointment with your health care provider, you may face several typical challenges: the visit may be rushed, you may not be thinking as clearly as usual because you are not feeling well, and you may remember an important question only after you have left. To help make your visits more informative, you should ask questions you have thought about beforehand. During the appointment, you should take the time to write down the answers, or you should bring someone with you who will write down the answers so that you can think about them later.

The questions that follow are reasonable to ask and show that you are actively involved in your health care. While your health care provider may give you an informational brochure to read later, it is also good to hear your health care provider's thoughts directly.

QUESTIONS ABOUT ADDITIONAL TESTS OR PROCEDURES

1. *Would you repeat (or write down) the name of the test or procedure?*

2. *What will this test or procedure tell you?*

3. *Can you explain how this test is done?*

4. *How soon do I need to have this test or procedure?*

5. *Are there other tests or procedures that could give similar information?*

6. *I know I will probably be given forms to sign that will describe a lot of the risks, but are there any risks that I should be concerned about with this recommended test or procedure?*

7. Do I have to do anything special before I have this test or procedure (such as not drink water, not eat, or not use body powder)?

8. How much will it hurt? (If your health care provider says you will have some "discomfort," ask what she or he means by that term.)

9. How can I make it easier for myself to take this test?

10. Will I get this test done here? If not, where will I get it done?

11. Do I need to make the appointment, or will your office do that?

12. How soon will I get the results?

13. Who will give me the results?

14. Should I call your office, or will you call me?

15. What happens if the results are positive?

QUESTIONS AFTER A DIAGNOSIS

1. Do you think the disease you have identified is causing me to feel the way I do?

2. What does that mean is happening to my body?

3. Is there a cure for this disease? Please explain your answer, whether it is yes or no.

4. What treatments are available?

5. Can you explain the risks and long-term benefits of the treatment?

6. What can I do to make the treatment most effective?

7. How soon do I need to make a decision about treatment?

8. Is there someone in your office who can talk to me about this? If I have questions later, whom should I call?

9. Where else can I get more information?

10. I have heard that there are clinical trials for some conditions. Do you think I should be part of a clinical trial (research study)?

QUESTIONS ABOUT SURGERY
ABOUT THE PROCEDURE

1. *Do I have to have surgery, or are there any nonsurgical options?*

2. *What would you expect to be different for me if I have this surgery?*

3. *Have there been problems with this type of surgery?*

4. *How successful is this surgery?*

5. *Which hospital is best for this surgery?*

6. *Where can I get a second opinion about the surgery I am considering?*

7. *If I go with your recommendation, who will actually be doing the surgery? If it is someone other than you, when will I meet that person?*

8. *How many times have you (or that person) done this surgery?*

9. *I know there are different kinds of anesthesia. Can you explain how they differ and which one you think would be best for me?*

10. *I know it is important to meet the anesthesiologist before my surgery. When will I meet her or him?*

11. *How long will the actual surgery take?*

12. *Will the person I designate as my health care advocate be kept informed about the progress of my surgery while it is under way and, afterward, the result of the surgery?*

13. *Whom can I ask whether my health insurance will cover all aspects of the surgery—the pre–hospital admission tests, the hospital stay, the surgeons and anesthesiologists, the rehabilitative services, and so on?*

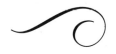

ABOUT RECOVERY AFTER SURGERY

1. *How long after the surgery will I have to stay in the hospital?*

2. *After the surgery, how much pain will I have?*

3. *Will I be given medicines to take at home?*

4. *Will I be able to go home after the surgery, or will I probably need additional care elsewhere? If I cannot go directly home, where will I go, and when will I be able to go home?*

5. *Will I be able to drive home? If not, how long will it be before I can drive?*

6. *When I go home, will I need*

   - *Someone to help me with my daily activities?* Yes No

   - *Special food?* Yes No

   - *Special equipment?* Yes No

7. *When I am home, will I be able to*

   - *Go to the bathroom by myself?* Yes No *(If no, when could I?)*

   - *Shower by myself?* Yes No *(if no, when)*

   - *Go up and down stairs?* Yes No *(if no, when)*

   - *Cook for myself?* Yes No *(if no, when)*

8. *How soon after surgery will I be able to return to my daily routine?*

9. *When will I need to have follow-up appointments? Will those be with you or with someone else?*

More Resources

All of these resources are noncommercial ones, and they offer free information.

BEST FOR TALKING WITH A PERSON TO GET INFORMATION

The National Alliance for Hispanic Health has bilingual (English and Spanish) health promotion advisors who will send you free information and direct you to local clinics for services. They answer calls Monday through Friday, 9:00 a.m. to 6:00 p.m., Eastern Standard Time. For all health questions you can call toll-free, 1-866-783-2645 (1-866-Su Familia); or for information on prenatal care, call 1-800-504-7081.

BEST OVERALL WEBSITES FOR HEALTH INFORMATION

ENGLISH

- medlineplus.gov
- 4woman.gov *(limited materials in Spanish)*
- hispanichealth.org

SPANISH

- medlineplus.gov/spanish/
- hispanichealth.org

While you can search the Internet and get lots of information, much of it is not accurate, and sometimes what seems like "information" is a promotion for a specific product or procedure, or an attempt to get your personal information. Very often it is difficult to tell who is actually making the information available to you. When it comes to the health of women, we all—and especially Latinas—need to carefully review information we find online.

The following resources, provided by topic, should help you get helpful, specific, reliable information. Please let me know if you come across better sources of information.

Specific Places to Call

Air Quality

Indoor Air Quality Information Clearinghouse (IAQINFO)
1-800-438-4318/no Spanish line
This is the best hotline for information on air quality. This organization makes referrals to other local government agencies. You may call on Monday through Friday, 10 a.m. to 4 p.m. No Spanish speakers are available.

Food and Food-Borne Illnesses

USDA Hotline 1-800-535-4555/Spanish menu option
This hotline is for basic information and reporting problems about meat, poultry, and processed egg products. Extensive information is available over the phone, and referrals can be made to online and downloadable information. You may call on Monday through Friday, 10:00 a.m. to 4:00 p.m.

CDC Hotline • 1-800-232-4636/Spanish menu option
If you or someone you know becomes ill, or if you would like information on food-borne illnesses, you can call this number, which is available twenty-four hours a day, seven days a week.

FDA Safefood Hotline • 1-888-723-3366/no Spanish
This hotline provides information on foods (except red meat, poultry, and processed eggs), and the staff can connect you to the proper authorities for issues related to the mishandling of food. The FDA will

send you fact sheets on what safe food is and how to keep it safe, as well as direct you to online information and make referrals. You may call on Monday through Friday, 10:00 a.m. to 4:00 p.m.

GENETICS INFORMATION

GENETICS AND RARE DISEASES INFORMATION CENTER
1-888-205-2311 TTY: 1-888-205-3223/Spanish menu option
This toll-free phone line is available from 12:00 p.m. to 6:00 p.m., Monday through Friday, Eastern Standard Time.

WATER

SAFE DRINKING WATER HOTLINE (EPA)
1-800-426-4791/Spanish menu option
The staff of this hotline can address your concerns about annual water quality reports, household wells, public drinking-water systems, local drinking-water quality, drinking-water standards, source-water protection; large-capacity residential septic systems, commercial and industrial septic systems, injection wells, and drainage wells. You may call on Monday through Friday, 10:00 a.m. to 4:00 p.m.

STORET WATER QUALITY SYSTEM HOTLINE
1-800-424-9067/no Spanish
This hotline keeps information through the Storet water-data system. Unless you have a specific question (as in, "Please give me information on lead levels in the water of Los Angeles during 2006), the staff will transfer you to a regional number answered by the specific person who handles the information for that region. Be aware that a regional number you are transferred to may not be a toll-free number, so there may be a charge for your call. You may call on Monday through Friday, 10:00 a.m. to 4:30 p.m.

WEBSITES ON SPECIAL TOPICS

HOSPITALS: HOW TO COMPARE THEM

CENTER FOR MEDICAID AND MEDICARE SERVICES (CMS)
www.hospitalcompare.hhs.gov
This government-sponsored website provides information on how well hospitals care for patients with certain medical conditions or surgical procedures. It also has results from a survey of patients about the quality of care they received during a recent hospital stay.

THE COMMONWEALTH FOUNDATION
www.WhyNotTheBest.org
This foundation-sponsored website provides information on hospitals and allows you to compare a hospital against its peers.

MEDICATIONS

PHYSICIANS' DESK REFERENCE
www.pdrhealth.com
This website, offered by the publishers of Physicians' Desk Reference provides extensive information about available medications. Through an "interaction checker," it can help you understand whether there are medications interactions that may be of concern. It also includes information on alternative medicines and treatment options.

NANOTECHNOLOGY

NATIONAL INSTITUTES OF HEALTH—NANOMEDICINE
nihroadmap.nih.gov/nanomedicine/
From this website you can subscribe to the NIH's nanomedicine e-mail list. It also has links to NIH nanoscience and nano-technology information.

FOOD AND DRUG ADMINISTRATION—NANOTECHNOLOGY
www.fda.gov/nanotechnology/
This website provides an overview of the July 2007 FDA
Nanotechnology Task Force Report. It also has links to recent consumer
articles and other federal agencies involved in nanotechnology.

POSITIVE PSYCHOLOGY

DR. MARTIN SELIGMAN, UNIVERSITY OF PENNSYLVANIA
www.authentichappiness.org
This is the website for Dr. Martin Seligman, the director of the
University of Pennsylvania's Positive Psychology Center and the founder
of the positive psychology field. This site has tests you can take,
resources, and newsletters.

SLEEP

NATIONAL SLEEP FOUNDATION
www.sleepfoundation.org
This foundation is dedicated to improving the quality of life for
Americans who suffer from sleep problems and disorders.

CENTERS FOR DISEASE CONTROL
www.cdc.gov/sleep/hygiene.htm
The CDC offers tips on how to get regular sleep.

WATER (DRINKING)

ENVIRONMENTAL PROTECTION AGENCY
www.epa.gov/ow
The EPA Office of Water's website contains information on drinking-
water laws and regulations, and other resources you can order.

ACKNOWLEDGMENTS

MAKING THIS BOOK POSSIBLE TOOK THE SUPPORT AND belief of many people. Janet Goldstein, my editor, helped me shape this book into a reality. A special thanks goes to the entire team at Newmarket Press for their enthusiasm and commitment to this book: Esther Margolis, Heidi Sachner, Keith Hollaman, and Harry Burton. Newmarket is what is best about publishing and its future. There are also key members of my staff at the National Alliance for Hispanic Health who were always helpful and have committed their professional lives to making life better for everybody: Kevin Adams, Brenda Chase, Magdalena Castro-Lewis, Marcela Gaitan, Edgar Gil, Eliana Loveluck, Demitria Morrison, Hazel Moss, Concha Orozco, and Melissa Perez.

To keep my mind refreshed and to provide the emotional support I needed for my life and my writing, I depended on my very special and brilliant *amigas* and *comadres* (Lourdes Baezconde-Garbanati, Carolyn Curiel, Polly Gault, Ileana Herrell, Margaret Heckler, Sheila Raviv, Carolina Reyes, Esther Sciammarella, and Amanda Spivey); daily contact with Adolph Falcon, my friend and colleague for nearly twenty-five years; Cynthia A. Telles, my life sister; my wonderful daughter, Elizabeth Delgado Steo, who reminds me that our children truly are our legacy and a blessing; and my husband, Mark Steo, who is always showing me that marriage is about love and joy.

Finally, there are those who helped shape my life and with whom I can no longer make new memories: Deborah Helvarg; Henrietta Villasecusa; and, of course, my very special and incredible mom, Lucy Delgado. Mom, Deborah, and Henrietta may be gone, but their spirits continue to teach and strengthen me each and every day. Their love is a part of my heart, and this book is offered from my heart to you.

INDEX

ABOUT THE AUTHOR

JANE L. DELGADO, Ph.D., M.S., author of *The Latina Guide to Health: Consejos and Caring Answers*, is President and Chief Executive Officer of the National Alliance for Hispanic Health ("the Alliance"), the nation's largest organization of health and human service providers to Hispanics. She was recognized by *WebMD* as one of its four Health Heroes of 2008 for her dedication and resilience in advocacy, among many other awards and honors, including the 2007 *People En Español* 100 Influentials in the Hemisphere and the 2005 Hispanic Heritage Foundation Award for Education.

A practicing clinical psychologist, Dr. Delgado joined the Alliance in 1985 after serving in the Immediate Office of the Secretary of the U.S. Department of Health and Human Services (DHHS), where she became a key force in the development of the landmark "Report of the Secretary's Task Force on Black and Minority Health."

At the Alliance, Dr. Delgado oversees the national staff as well as field operations throughout the United States, Puerto Rico, and the District of Columbia. She is also a trustee of the Kresge Foundation, Lovelace Respiratory Research Institute, the U.S. Soccer Foundation, Northern Virginia Health Foundation, and the Health Foundation for the Americas, and serves on the national advisory councils for the Paul G. Rogers Society for Global Health Research and on the National Board of Mrs. Rosalyn Carter's Task Force on Mental Health.

Dr. Delgado received her M.A. in Psychology from New York University in 1975. In 1981 she was awarded a Ph.D. in clinical psychology from SUNY Stony Brook and an M.S. in Urban and Policy Sciences from the W. Averell Harriman School of Urban and Policy Sciences. She lives in Washington, D.C., with her husband, Mark, and daughter, Elizabeth.

Founded in 1973, **The National Alliance for Hispanic Health** is the foremost science-based source of information and trusted advocate for the health of Hispanics. The Alliance represents local community agencies serving more than 15 million persons each year, and national organizations serving over 100 million persons, making a daily difference in the lives of Hispanic communities and families.

The Health Foundation for the Americas (HFA) supports the work and mission of the National Alliance for Hispanic Health, and seeks individuals, companies, agencies, foundations, and sponsors to help support its programs to improve the quality of healthcare for all, which includes providing timely and trusted bilingual health information. Every year HFA supports programs to improve health for all by helping secure clean air to breathe, clean water to drink, safe places to play, and healthy food to eat. HFA and the Alliance help those without healthcare gain access to free and low-cost services where they live and improve the quality of healthcare. The programs put new health technology to work in communities, provide millions of dollars in science and health career scholarships, and conduct the research and advocacy that is transforming health.

Dr. Delgado's book *The Latina Guide to Health: Consejos and Caring Answers* is published simultaneously in English- and Spanish-language editions by Newmarket Press. The author is donating all royalties from the Spanish edition to The Health Foundation for the Americas (HFA).

You can be a part of this extraordinary mission of health and well-being. To learn more about the Alliance or the HFA, visit www.hispanichealth.org or www.healthyamericas.org.